THE EDGE AND BEYOND

2ND EDITION

A JOURNEY FOR PERSONAL SELF-DISCOVERY AWAKENING AND HEALING

LANCE J. MORRIS, ND

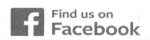
Find us on Facebook

Copyright © 2010 by Lance J. Morris ND

Copyright © 2nd Edition 2014

Published by Third-Eye Awake Press
1601 N. Tucson Blvd #37
Tucson, AZ 85716

Library of Congress Cataloging-in-Publication Data:

Morris, Lance J.

The Edge and Beyond: A Journey for
Personal Self-Discovery,
Awakening and Healing
Lance J. Morris ND
2nd.Ed
p. cm. Index
Includes bibliographical references and index
Library of Congress control number: 2013957539
ISBN 978-0-9837941-1-0

1. Spirituality 2. Self-Help 3. Health
4. Energy Medicine 5. Naturopathy
6. Physics (New Thought) I. Title

Printed in USA

CONTENTS

BLANK NOTES PAGE

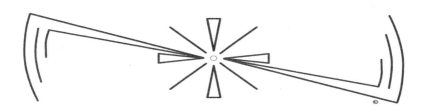

ACKNOWLEDGEMENTS

I want to humbly thank my parents for their great gift of courage and sacrifice to allow me into the world, through them. I want to especially thank my sister Jaye, my greatest ally, who knows and understands me better than anyone. Her keen insight and intuition is flawless and from which I still have much to learn. Without her tireless effort, as my right hand editor, this book would still be on the drawing table. To my wife and sons who are my greatest teachers, challenge and joy. To my spiritual brother and co-mentor Michael Katz. Thank you for your tolerance and love to let me wake up and embrace our gem stone allies. Our mirrors shine bright for each other. To Stella Ede, thank you for helping the rewrite of the book's introduction and beginning headings. Heartfelt gratitude to Sheri Herrera de Frey for her impeccable sense of grammar and the courage and commitment to nitpick every sentence of this book, which helped me refine details, definitions and linkages to improve this 2nd edition. Your contributions were priceless.

Thank you to all the plants and animals. A heartfelt appreciation to cats for their special and unique role in bringing *RST*: Resonant Sound Therapy to this dimension. Love to mother Earth and father sky. To all my relations, friends, patients and colleagues that have looked over my shoulder as *RST, RMM*: Resonant Movement Meditation and this book have developed with encouragement and anticipation, the wait is over. To all my spiritual teachers and guides from the physical and non-physical realms, thank you so much for your patience, unconditional love and willingness to hang in there with me. I, like you, have chosen the path of service; to BE a voice and vehicle for the divine will, to wake up as one, as many, in the moment, to *The Edge and Beyond*.

FORWARD

Gary E. Schwartz, PhD

Professor of Psychology, Medicine, Neurology, Psychiatry and Surgery, and Director, Laboratory for Advances in Consciousness and Health, University of Arizona. His books include *The Afterlife Experiments, The G.O.D. Experiments, The Energy Healing Experiments,* and *The Sacred Promise.*

It has been said that many have been called but few will be chosen. I hold the space that all have been called and the time is NOW!

Lance J. Morris, ND

Humanity is at a crossroads. We can continue to behave as we have in the past and destroy ourselves and the planet in the process, or we can choose to transform our habits, to actualize our higher potential, and contribute to healing ourselves and the world.

This urgent message is coming from many quarters — from ancient cultures and native peoples, through contemporary mystics and new age thinkers, to professional writers, scientists and celebrity entertainers. Novelists like William Gladstone have fictionalized this possibility in *The Twelve.*

Systems scientists like Dr. Erwin Laszlo have documented this opportunity in *WorldShift 2012,* or as presented in my book *The Sacred Promise.*

Entertainers like the late Michael Jackson – who wrote the visionary song, *We are the World* – creatively express this urgency in *This Is It*. Though our modes of communication are different – spanning fiction and story-telling, basic and applied research, music and dance – the core message of the pressing need for our personal and collective awakening and transforming is the same.

How are we to make sense of all this? And what can we do as individuals to contribute to this emerging transformation? *The Edge and Beyond* provides what Dr. Lance Morris, the visionary author of this book, calls a *primer for the personal actualization of this state*.

What is this state? According to Dr. Morris, the state involves the recognition that not only are we co-creators with the *Source* of All that is, but that we all have the power within for *Tapping the Source* as revealed in William Gladstone and colleague's *how to* book of this title.

According to Dr. Morris, *our co-creation is manifest as a channel or conduit of the divine.* He says that this is, *a function of thy will, not my will.*

We can find and be a vehicle for this as we approach and move through the last membrane of the space-time continuum, to The Edge and Beyond.

The Edge and Beyond combines philosophy and basic science with ancient and contemporary healing practices – including an innovative healing technique developed by Dr. Morris called *RST: Resonant Sound Therapy.*

He reveals an exciting new framework for achieving scientific and personal integration and unification. *The Edge and Beyond* is more than just a highly reader friendly book; it is informative and insightful on the one hand, and inspirational and playful on the other.

This is the kind of book which you will read from cover to cover, and then reread (and even reread again).

Certain books are so easy to digest on first reading yet provide expanded nourishment upon rereading.

Dr. Morris's subtitle, *A Journey for Personal Self-Discovery, Awakening, and Healing* is accurate and meaningful.

This is a book which contains practical information all of us can learn to employ in our daily lives. The second edition brings a level of increased clarity, detail to definition and more refined linkages, with over a hundred and fifty pages of new material.

His conclusions of a *Unified Field Theory* brings physics out of the clouds into everyday life. The astounding, yet practical connections between *fascia,* sound, frequencies, the *mobius* of infinity, the *double helix* of DNA, the *Big Bang, Cosmic Inflation, String Theory,* the Singularity of Black Holes and faster than light speed travel, offer a personal tool box to access dimensions beyond what Dr. Morris calls *STEM; space-time, energy* and *matter.* Hold on for a wild and fabulous ride!

I asked Dr. Morris to provide me with a visionary statement of what he wished for this book. His last paragraph says it all, and I invite you to partake of this extraordinary journey with his words in mind:

We are on a critical cusp. The choice is ours. We can implode or we can transcend. We have been here before. Throughout history this cycle is repeated time and again. This book is a wakeup call. All over this planet messengers have been seeded to bring different parts of this information into the public domain. The time is now. We are the ones we have been waiting for.

It is our choice to succumb to our own negative images, feelings and mental projections or to awaken triumphant, to transcend to The Edge and Beyond. It has been said that many have been called but few will be chosen. I hold the space that all have been called and the time is NOW!

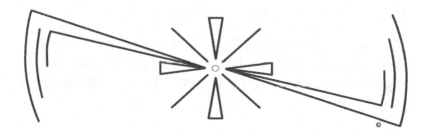

INTRODUCTION

Welcome to *The Edge and Beyond*. There are no accidents and no coincidences. This statement is not intended to support a deterministic view of our lives or existence. It is to acknowledge our capacity to perceive *patterns* and use *free will* to enter into a *cause* or effect relationship with the pattern. If you have picked up this book, perhaps you are ready. Ready for what, you might ask? To *be* ready to clarify, expand and reinforce your own unique personal world view.

This book is intended to be used as a mirror to help you solidify and contract, then liquefy and expand your personal view or perception of yourself and your world. I will bring you on a journey of discovery and awakening from the world of atoms, to the world of stars, to the worlds between worlds, from the finite to the infinite and beyond.

I offer a framework in which our perceptions and experiences can be seen and identified within the context of a value system: good or better than; bad or worse than. This value system is a projection and perception derived from our familial, linguistic, social and cultural upbringing and heritage. Such a value system limits and binds us.

Our awareness and identification of self, with value systems, is a critical step in our awakening journey. It allows us to clearly see a defined limit or edge.

As we find these clear limits and edges, it is our birthright and spiritual imperative to systematically pierce them moving into an ever expanding and transcendent awareness.

I bring many edges into clear focus, then pierce them. It is my intention to help my readers learn to find, then pierce, their own edges or limits. For some this may parallel my own journey, and for others, it may lead them into very different places. I personally find this exciting and comforting.

I encourage and support our ability to mutually embrace each other and revel in our unique individual perceptions and differences.

As we move from one edge, then beyond, to another edge, then beyond, through all edges or limits and beyond, we eventually enter a value-free system which acts to equalize all perceptions and experiences. The *key* to *being cause* is not derived from any perception or experience directly; neither does our belief, nor conviction in the truth or correctness of our perception or experience control nor create *cause.*

The *key* to *being cause* is the utilization of our *free will* choice, with any and all perceptions and experiences, to be neutral or *unconditional.* This requires not bringing any charged negative emotions or mental value judgments to any specific perception or experience. Any charged negative emotions or judgments make us the *effect* of our own causation.

As we are waking up, charged emotions and judgments inevitably surface. This is natural. Don't try to stop them or shut them off but rather practice observing them and identifying where, or to what, any charge or judgment is linked or attached. Create a *mock-up,* as an internal visual image replaying the perception or experience as *neutral.* The more we practice, the easier it gets.

We realize that perceptions and experiences offer the opportunity for daily practice in the art of reacting or not reacting. From this position, our choices and actions come from our awareness and understanding of *cause* and *effect*. Our choices and actions are no longer linked or derived from a relativistic moral or ethical value standard. We are freed from the influence of either internal or external judgments projected as shame, blame or guilt. Our choice is now guided by intuition or divine intent.

Throughout this book, I share many generalized and personal perceptions and views. These perceptions and views contract (solidify) and alternately expand (liquefy) our awareness and consciousness. This book is filled with paradoxes. It is through paradox that we can personally discover how to reconcile seemingly different perceptions or views of the same thing, not as right or wrong, but as pieces of a greater whole.

Think of this book as a road map to refine, expand and clarify your own unique perceptions and world views. I illuminate how to use paradox as a tool in this *process* to personally contract and expand your perception and view into an ever larger, wider, and more encompassing perspective. As this perceptual expansion occurs, a wonderful and natural side effect is that we become more understanding, tolerant, accepting and unconditionally loving, both to ourselves and others.

The term *process* refers to the detailed specifics of how to find and utilize the road map. Understanding and mastering *process* is the key to everything. What comes out of *process* as things or results are secondary.

Culturally, we are prone to place things and results as primary. *Process* as the skill or tool set necessary to make a thing or have an outcome is sustainable, useful and practical. Its *essence* is imperishable, while that which *process* makes, or its results, are impermanent and perishable.

At this point in my book, since this is only the introduction, I beseech my readers to take a deep breath, suspend judgment at this early stage, and enjoy a journey of self-discovery. I have been a student and seeker my whole life. This book is an expression of many universal threads that connect us as one. Through personal stories, examples and insights, I weave a cohesive story of our common journey. This journey leads to many paths, many teachers, and many experiences.

As a practicing Naturopathic physician since 1985, I have been privileged to discover and re-awaken in myself and others the fascial membrane. This membrane surrounds every part of the body and plays a critical role in maintaining health and expanding consciousness. This book is about finding and identifying *forms*, placing them in a contextual framework, mastering them, and then releasing them to move into the *formless*.

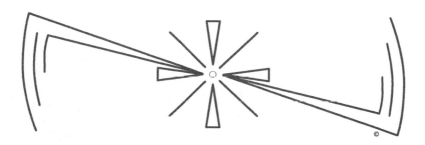

My personal and professional discoveries, combined with the awakening and understanding of what the fascial membrane is, have led to the development of a bio-energetic therapy I call *Resonant Sound Therapy (RST)* and *Resonant Movement Meditation (RMM)*.

This therapy and meditative practice is referred to throughout the book, it is the medium through which my personal awareness and insights have sprung. Welcome to my world and hang on!

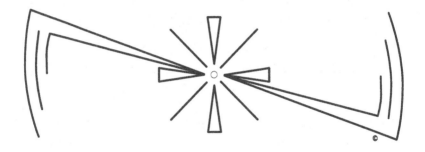

NOTE FROM THE AUTHOR

You may read this book, in the traditional way, from left to right and from beginning to end. I suggest an alternative for your consideration.

First, read the forward and introduction in the normal linear fashion. After that, any time you pick up this book, relax, clear your head, open your heart and take a few deep breaths. Open the book randomly, *holding the space* for the universe or the divine to guide or direct you. Don't project or intend any specific outcome, choose to trust the universe to fill in the details for you. A truly amazing and remarkable result happens when we stop pushing the door from the inside out with our *body, ego, mind* and *identity* and allow the door to open inwardly, to be filled by universal, divine intent.

Opening the book randomly, read one bold-type title and contents, which can be one paragraph to a few pages. There are no chapters in this book, each bold-type title stands as a complete independent unit of information. From that point in the book you can read additional bold titles either to the right or the left. As this is done, an increase in information and clarity around the initial topic will develop.

This formatting was intentional on my part to offer a unique method to read the material. It is a mirror reflection of a natural and deeper *process* whereby we are all waking up and connecting the dots in an ever expanding sphere from a central core.

This reading *process,* done with friends, family or a discussion group can be entertaining and challenging. Read a bold title out loud and engage in a dialogue or discussion about the material, then pass it on to the next person and repeat the *process.*

Cause versus Effect

When we are *cause*, we control our destiny. When we are *effect*, destiny controls us. What does it mean in the human experience to *solidify* and *contract*, or to *liquefy* and *expand* our awareness and beliefs? How are our perceptions of *less than, more than, better than,* and *worse than* shaping our reality? Exploring these concepts will bring enhanced understanding of the *cause* and *effect* relationship of controlling or being controlled by our destiny. These concepts are important building blocks for the material that is presented throughout the book; they also lay the foundation for *Resonant Sound Therapy (RST)* and *Resonant Movement Meditation (RMM)*. *RST* is a bio-energetic healing therapy using resonant vocal tones from the therapist and patient simultaneously. Therapeutic touch, in a circular rhythmic motion, is concurrently utilized. *RMM* integrates vocal sound and circular rhythmic motion by an individual to maintain and potentiate *RST* therapy.

Throughout this book there are occasions when I use specific words or terms framed in different or unusual ways or with unique definitions. These different framings or definitions are derived from my personal experiences, awareness, and perception using *Resonant Sound Therapy (RST) and Resonant Movement Meditation (RMM)* for myself or with my patients. By taking the framing, context or definition I suggest, at face value, a greater depth of clarity and understanding will *be* realized.

If the words or terms used are approached from the perspective of standard definitions, it will reduce, rather than enhance, understanding.

I share information and make statements without qualifiers. They are presented as being true or factual. Much of the information I share, or statements I make, may not be regarded as *common knowledge* or be readily accepted as accurate or true. The axioms: *question authority, question reality or question everything* are guiding principles I apply and advocate for my readers. So-called *common* or *standard knowledge* may be anything but true or accurate. This has been demonstrated and proven time and time again. I admonish my readers to be mindful about strongly defending any *common knowledge, dogma* or seeming *truth.* Shared information and statements are based on my authentic personal experience, perception and awareness. They are intended to be fun, challenging, and thought provoking. They are not intended to be authoritative or incendiary.

In my personal awakening journey, one of my lessons in the *process* of developing and expanding perception and awareness is: *every time I come to believe or think that I have some definitive, incontestable or absolute truth, the universe or spirit, with flawless precision, has always demonstrated otherwise.* This is a profoundly humbling yet balancing experience. This lesson has led to a fundamental concept: *from the contracted to the expanded, to the contracted, to the more expanded. The expanded does not negate the contracted, it is merely additive.*

Not *The Truth,* but rather *A Truth,* are pieces that link together in an ever widening, expanding *sphere.* All perceived truth is subject to change or modification. This is a journey from the finite to the infinite, to *The Edge and Beyond.*

To Solidify or Liquefy

To solidify an edge creates a boundary that defines a *clear limit.* It is like the contents within a box which are known and finite. This solidified space may be perceived as comforting and secure. We know what we know, and we know that we know it. A limit, by definition, is *less than.*

To liquefy an edge, its boundary is fluid or in flux. This liquefaction defines an *unclear limit.* There is no definitive box and the contents may be infinite. This liquefied space, or unclear limit, may be perceived as uncomfortable and insecure. A swaddled or tightly wrapped baby, held against a warm body with an audible heartbeat, feels more secure than a naked baby left on the top of a bed.

An unclear limit, by definition, is *more than. More than* is not better and *less than* is not worse. The mind may frame the perception of *more* as better and *less* as worse. Specific situations or circumstances support personal experience and interpretation to validate a directional value judgment. If a solid box and its contents are perceived as more comfortable and secure, *less than* may be better. Personal perception is of paramount importance.

So-called facts or truth may or may not support personal perception. The way things are perceived, is in fact, the way they are. That is, the way they are to us. Perception may be deemed inaccurate or incorrect based on some standard of external authority agreed upon by a majority of people. This standardized information may neither be true or accurate. From the perspective of a limited box of perception, the way something is perceived is valid, correct and true, regardless of any other perceived or projected truths from any other source.

When *common belief* was the Earth was flat, we were confident of our box of perception and its contents. We felt stable and secure. When we were challenged in this belief and offered a new paradigm that the world was round, this made us feel unstable and insecure. This insecurity supported the misuse of authority to kill or imprison those who would not recant this new seemingly false paradigm. We can look back at this historic juncture and smile at our own foolishness in clinging to a false belief. The world perceived as flat, was a limited perceptual box. Within the border or boundary of personal perceptual verification, based solely on reliance of the five human senses of seeing, hearing, smelling, tasting and touching, the proof of the flatness of Earth continues to remain fundamentally self-evident.

Knowing the world is round, the perception of flatness *is less than* and defines a more limited perceptual box. How do we know that the world is round?

This awareness and belief is not obvious as a function of utilization of our five human senses in isolation. It is primarily through tools of mathematics and physics, combined with telescopes and satellite pictures which scientists use to readily and authoritatively state the fact of the world as round. The world perceived as round is a larger perceptual box. Within its own border or boundary of perceptual and cognitive verification or proof, it seems true. This truth relies on information that is not purely perceptual, it includes externally derived abstract data that frames it as a seeming truth. This seeming truth is expanded; it is *more than.* It may be perceived that more is better. Better or worse is always framed in a *context* in which we place a linear value judgment or graduated perception of worth on a thing or idea.

What if the world as round can also be framed as a piece of an even larger and greater truth? From this perspective, the world as round becomes a limited perceptual box as well. It is *less than.* Then what is *The Truth?* You might be thinking, *now wait a minute! The Earth is round is a clear scientific fact. You can't try to compare our previously erroneous perception of the Earth as flat with our current, correct and accurate perception that the Earth is round. This is uncontestable.* Really? When people believed the Earth was flat, they were just as confident about the integrity of that truth, and their proof of it, as we are confident today about the integrity and truth that the world is round. The world as round is an expanded perception relative to the world as flat.

An exciting and amazing possibility is that the world is much more than either of these two superficial physical qualities.

The Plus Factor

The *plus factor* introduces the premise that anything that we see, perceive, interpret or utilize has an additive component. This *process* identifies that anything framed as *The Way* or the *absolute* correct perception and interpretation is limited. It is limited because there is no ability to add to it; there is no *plus factor.* Framing anything that we see, perceive, interpret or utilize as *A Way* allows the addition of a *plus factor.* The challenge is to discover and recognize the *plus factor* in your own life. This allows us to step out of our *ego,* which is part of our projected construct of self-identification.

This frees us from the tyranny of having to *be right.* We can relax in the confidence that our awareness, perceptions and interpretations usually represent a *contracted and limited* box. This allows us to *be humble* and remember, *the more we know, the more we know* and paradoxically, *the more we know, the less we know.* The excessive value we assign to a perception or thing binds or limits our ability to let it go and embrace the *plus factor.*

That which creates a value system is conditional, and that which is value free is *unconditional.* Conditional means there are conditions. Conditions define a clear limit. A clear limit is a box, it is *less than.* Unconditional means there are no conditions.

Unconditional defines an unclear limit. An unclear limit has no box, it is *more than*. Between the conditional and the unconditional are a series of bigger and bigger perceptual boxes. At the transition cusp of the conditional to the *unconditional*, the last box is pierced. We have arrived at the final edge and are ready to enter the great beyond.

Value free is not devoid of value. It is only devoid of our limited contextual framework from which we give value to a person, place, thing, feeling or thought. This value is relative to perceptions or projections of a theoretical and relativistic good, bad, right or wrong. This value is derived from our linguistic, familial, social, cultural, religious, political and moral indoctrination.

Existence has a cyclical quality. This cyclical nature is expressed through many variable levels of perception and reality. One aspect characterized through many levels is an alternating expansion and contraction, then contraction and expansion. Each cycle of contraction and expansion is less contractive and more expansive. As each cycle expands, prior perceptions or views or limits still remain valid and true but now there is a broader ever expanding perceptual component. This expanded perception never negates or limits anything, it is always additive.

As this expansion occurs, we enter into the mysterious realm of paradox. A paradox is simply two different views or perceptions of the same thing that on the surface seem to be in conflict, contradict, or negate each other, while in fact, they do not.

Paradoxes function to contract (solidify) our perception and expand (liquefy) it. As we see and touch a pencil it is perceived as solid and smooth. A pencil examined under a microscope is porous and rough. At the atomic level, the pencil has no solidity, it is pure energy. This illustrates our ability to expand, contract and expand even more.

The truth about the pencil at all levels is true. The expanded levels do not negate the contracted levels, the expanded levels are just additive. The expanded or additive level, being *more than*, may seem on the surface, to be *better than*. This projection of value, by definition, is derived from a conditional state. A pencil is solid and not solid at the same time. This is a statement of fact, neither being better nor worse than the other.

Owning more than one house, is *more than*. On the surface, this *more than* may seem better. The perception of *more than* is accurate, however, the placing of a value of *better than* is a projection. Such a projection may have no basis in reality. If the mortgage payments and maintenance on additional properties cannot be met, the perception and reality may be that *more is less*, or *more is worse than*. The ability to perceive this expanded perceptual framing now becomes obvious, as it relates to a variety of personal experiences or situations.

To Suspend Judgment

Practice *suspending judgment.* This is to refrain from placing a value on anything. Suspension of judgment opens a space for a more expansive state of *being*.

Be calm, centered, and relaxed, don't project negative feelings or judgments, and just allow awareness to pass the filter censure of the *mind-brain*. The *process* of expanding and contracting awareness and perception moves us in and out of our comfort zone and across defined and undefined limits. This may induce unpleasant physical, emotional or mental reactions. Understanding and expecting these reactions is a useful barometer to evaluate our state of *being* expanded and unconditional, versus contracted and conditional. *Being* unconditional allows us to *be* less reactive. As consciousness and awareness continues to expand *beingness* is actualized and the joy of the moment is realized.

The concept of the *mind-brain* stems from the question: Is consciousness or mind, encased in, and created by, the action of our body's brain exclusively, or is the mind independent of the body? Scientists, such as neurophysiologists, contend that the mind only exists in the physical brain. The foundation for this theoretical belief is associated with observations at the time of death of the physical body. Physical evidence supports brain death being concurrent with the death of the body.

Can this same correlation be made between the brain and the mind? Using observation coupled with logic an absolute deterministic theory, linking physical brain death with mind death, appears to have a scientific basis. A serious reader, willing to actively apply the tools and techniques presented here, can personally resolve the *mind-brain* question for themselves through direct experience.

A working title of this book was *Perfect Blueprint-Beyond Perfection*. Perfection is a solidification. The edge or boundary is clearly marked.

When the edge is clearly marked, then a limit has been identified. A limit by definition is *less than*. Perfection is an abstract concept created by mind. It is framed in a context that requires us to perceive, and then place, an emotional charge or projected value on a person, place, thing, feeling or thought. Perfection is not perfect. That which is perfect *is* beyond perfection. This is a paradox. Perfection is a *form*. A *form* has shape and clear boundaries. A *form* defines a limit. A *form* takes the shape of a person, place, thing, feeling or thought. A philosophy, concept, theory, ideology or religion is a *form*.

A working subtitle was; *The Form is not the Way, the Way is the Way, a Path Beyond Perfection*. To find the way, to find the formless, we use and master many forms along the path. The forms can point or lead to the way.

This book offers many tools and techniques (forms) to offer the opportunity to expand and contract, until we stop expansion or contraction. At this juncture, we enter into the formless or liquefied state, to the last identifiable membrane, through the final edge, into the beyond.

Mind and language are forms that help along the way. Let them go, to just *be*. The condition of *being* or *being formless* is a state of *being pure cause*. As *cause*, we are in control, the masters of our destiny.

The state of *being cause* or in control is not mind driven, although on the surface it may seem this way. Forms are transitional. They are to be used, mastered, understood and released. How do we let both mind and language go?

From the perspective or view point of the mind this seems ludicrous, maybe even nonsensical. If we don't have mind or language then what do we have and how can it possibly be something of value, functional use or relevance? Here is another paradox. In this *process* we do not throw away the mind or language. We discover there is another place or perceptual level from which to receive information that is neither framed nor derived from the context or limited box of the mind.

We are Co-creators

We are co-creators. We co-create by holding images in our mind's eye coupled with feeling and intent. Some of these images are memories, while others are projections that are linked to possible future timelines. A memory is a remembering of a past experience.

The capacity for memory is a function of our brain's cortex. Memory helps us validate the existence and directional flow of time. In the moment that we are processing a memory, the only thing that we have of it, is our memory of it. Our mind, from the cortical part of the brain, may claim enough supporting evidence to have us accept the reality of the past as actually having happened. As we contract and expand and expand and contract that which we perceive as real, is true. The expanded does not negate the contracted, it is merely additive.

The past is real and true, and paradoxically, in the moment, its reality is nothing more than a memory. The only way the past has any influence or power over us is if we combine the image of a specific memory with a negative emotional charge and or mental projection judgment. The image, as a memory, is without charge. The image has no power.

The power of creation is not specific or restricted to any feeling *form*. We are free to use the presumed good, bad or neutral at will. When any of these feeling forms are conditioned or connected with value judgment, we become *effect*. As *effect* we become locked in a perpetual loop of repeating experiences. The intent of these experiences is to offer us an opportunity to *objectify* our awareness and perception and then overlay a neutral, non-reactive, unconditioned response. This specific *free will* choice, applied to any experience, ends the perpetual loop and we become *cause.* Experiences offer a window to see them as opportunities for growth and expanded awareness.

Experiences are part of the toolbox we utilize to break through all limits to ultimately transcend all value-judgment systems.

Even when the motive feelings are conditioned, we can use this power of creation to bring into our lives, as well as the lives of others, presumed good things. I say *presumed* due to the relative nature of our awareness and beliefs. This complex idea portends the axiom: *be careful what you wish for, you may just get it.* Why does this sound ominous?

The implication is that there may be negative, unforeseen ramifications to what we wish or project for ourselves or others. It clearly suggests a probable *cause* and *effect* relationship associated with our choices and actions.

We may believe, based on an identification with a *higher power,* moral or ethical reference that we should not only project presumed good things and outcomes for self or others but that there is actually a moral imperative to do so. This is a curious and egocentric human construct. The reader may discover a more expanded insight or awareness to guide them relative to personal future projections, toward self or others. Conditional feelings are the fuel that gives power to images that make us *effect*. As *effect,* destiny controls us.

One of the great paradoxes is that time, being its own paradox, is the medium through which we are eventually able to perceive the mechanics of our co-creative power.

Time plays a crucial role, as there is a linear relationship between the degree of expanded consciousness, relative to perception and understanding of *causation mechanics*, and the time interval between the manifestation of experiences that are repeating as *effect*. *Causation mechanics* refers to the mechanistic components or details of the *process* of functioning and manifesting as *cause* rather than *effect*. The greater our awareness of *causation mechanics*, the faster the cycles repeat and the easier they are to recognize. The less our awareness of *causation mechanics*, the slower the cycles repeat and the harder they are to recognize.

This may seem counter intuitive but it is none the less the way the universe teaches and guides us to wake up to our destiny as *cause.* Although the less we know and understand, the more we need to know and understand, paradoxically that which we need to know and understand is available to us only in proportion to how much we already know and understand.

The more technical a topic the more background information and education is necessary to comprehend it. You can't be a physician, engineer or physicist just because you want or wish it. You have to put in the time, work and study to achieve these goals.

If you want a line of credit from a bank you have to be credit worthy. The condition of being credit worthy takes time, discipline and proper fiscal management.

The laws that govern *process,* in the physical universe, are reflections of the laws governing *process* in the spiritual universe. The axiom, *as-above - so-below* is accurate and meaningful.

Feelings that are neutral and *unconditional* like joy, love, gratitude, fulfillment, contentment, serenity, harmony, or balance, are the fuel that give power to an image as *pure cause*, without *effect.* As *cause,* we control destiny. The power or intent we then imbue into an image-memory-projection with neutral feelings flows from within us out, from within us, out into manifestation.

As *cause,* that which manifests is *unconditional* and *indeterminate.* To actually be neutral or *unconditional*, image-feelings cannot be linked with any *attachment.*

Manifestation, as *cause,* must be *indeterminate,* rather than determinate. To *be indeterminate,* the specificity of details within an outcome or manifestation are not known, or only known as broad sweeping generalities. *Holding this space* with unclear boundaries, borders or defined limits allows *source,* or the divine, to fill in the specificity of details. Stop trying to fill in *all* the details driven by the mind's ego. This shuts out the divine.

By letting go and letting God, outcomes, and manifestations are derived from the expanded, more than, unconditional, unlimited *being* state.

That which is determinate, by definition is conditioned. Wants or desires are attachments to a specific projected image. If the image-projection is conditioned, it manifests as *effect.*

This manifestation, as *effect,* may be determinate. We have the ability to magnify attachment by adding additional negative feelings like sorrow or anger and thoughts like remorse or guilt, linked to the outcomes of our projected images. It is only when the projected image, either manifesting or not, is linked with negatively charged emotions and mental judgments, which are conditioned attachments that we remain bound in the perpetual loop of *effect.*

Any or all of these, so-called, neutral, *unconditional* feelings can be conditioned. If our joy, or any other feeling, is dependent on a specific person, place or thing then it is not *unconditional.*

Some feelings are conditioned by definition: lust, anger, greed, vanity or attachment in any *form*. Feelings can be conditioned or unconditioned. The criteria that makes this differentiation is our personal awareness, consciousness, *free will* and choice. No one, and nothing external to us, can define, predict or project this differentiation. This is a personal, internal *process*. An image-memory-projection with neutral feelings is supportive of an equilibrium state. The outcome of this type of image-feeling is *indeterminate* rather than determinate. The image-projection is not forced or controlled from the *mind-ego*; it is not self-seeking.

It is not projected from the perspective of *my will*, but rather it is a *surrender* into *thy will* or the divine will.

Paradoxically the *indeterminate* space is the transcendent space that allows us to *be cause* and not *effect*.

It is the paradox of gaining control by giving up control. In Western culture, the above premise of surrender or release of control is not only difficult to understand but also often considered undesirable due to our cultural fixation on *ego* gratification.

Faith is a Key

The primary function and purpose of *RST* and *RMM* is to re-establish the balanced flow of *Chi, life force, spirit* throughout the body. When this *life force* is in equilibrium the body heals itself. Since *Chi* or *spirit* travels through *fascia,* it is essential to understand what *fascia* is and how it works.

Fascia is the connective tissue membrane under our skin. It not only covers our muscles, but it surrounds every organ, nerve and blood vessel. *Fascia* is the only part of our body that is connected everywhere. As this membrane awakens, we discover through direct experience, that we are not the body, and that our body is only a shell. The body is a temporary dwelling place for the spark of consciousness, our essence, which is who we really are. Neither faith nor belief cause this awakening. Faith is a key. Like all keys it opens a lock that allows entrance into a previously inaccessible place.

My definition of faith: a state of *being* in which we completely suspend or stop any projection or judgment. We open our hearts and consciousness to the possibility that there is more to our lives and existence than is obvious. Our potential knowledge and awareness extends beyond what is perceived from superficial levels of perception, derived from our five primary physical senses. This key is an essential tool for us to use as we solidify, liquefy and expand our views and perceptions, to *be* more fully, and awaken to our greater consciousness.

It is through the fascial membrane that consciousness enters into the body at birth. The importance and function of the fascial membrane, in all its varied and remarkable contexts, is the foundation of the development of *RST* and *RMM*. In its natural state of equilibrium, *fascia* is permeable, giving our consciousness free access in and out of the body shell.

Acupuncture meridians and *chakras*, the bio-energetic vortices that are the non-physical master control centers for our physical, emotional, causal, mental, subconscious and spiritual bodies, are embedded in the fascial membrane. When *Chi*, *life force*, flows without restriction through all our meridians and *chakras* we remain in balance, physically, emotionally, mentally and spiritually.

Physical, emotional, and mental imbalances induce a twisting of the fascial membrane causing blockage of *Chi* flow. Blocked *Chi* is a disruption of the balanced positive and negative energy current of which *Chi* is composed.

Twisting of the fascial membrane causes a focal energetic anomaly which disrupts *Chi* flow. This leads to physical, emotional, or mental symptoms or imbalances and potential disease. This happens due to a physical injury or trauma. It also happens when we engage an image in our mind's eye, coupled with a negative or conditioned emotional charge. Additionally, we twist *fascia* and block *Chi* by projecting any opinion or judgment, whether toward self or outside of self, toward people, places, things or thoughts.

The body viewed as a container has definitive edges. The discovery of self as *be-mi;* a *body* and *ego*, as well as a *mind* and *identity* comes through the refinement of our five primary senses of touch, hearing, sight, taste and smell combined with the cortical parts of our brain.

The senses and cortex act as a protective barrier to keep us from awakening and reaching or experiencing our existence as more than a body or *mind-brain*.

The cortex allows us to perceive and place ourselves in *space-time*. We can remember the past and project images into the future. Refinement of the five primary senses, combined with cortical functions of memory and projection, is how and why we make and link negative emotional charges that torque *fascia*.

Torqued *fascia*, blocking *Chi*, manifests physical, emotional, mental, subconscious, and spiritual symptoms or diseases.

Our senses and cortex are *forms;* they define a boundary or limit. They are essential tools we use to contract and expand, contract and expand more.

They bind and limit us, and as *forms*, they point to *the way* which is unbound and limitless. This boundless, expansive path is not found with our senses or cortex. Our senses and cortex act as a bridge for us to pass over or through in order to enter the *formless-limitless* realm.

Mathematics is a Pure Universal Language

Mathematics is a pure universal language. Regardless of which spoken language is utilized, communication using numbers is instant, with full mutual understanding. Because of this understanding, humans are transmitting numeric signals into space seeking a response from other intelligent life forms.

Math is often referred to as *the language of the universe.* Math is used to describe or enhance the meaning or understanding of sound or music.

There is a natural translational relationship between sound and math. Essential properties of *RST* include resonance and harmonics. We experience these properties by listening to sounds or through the induction of vocal sounds used in *RST*. Mathematics is another medium through which the properties of resonance and harmonics may be described or understood.

Math is a tool to enhance understanding the nature of the universe and existence. We live in a relative universe filled with paradox. An elegant and simple mathematical example or explanation of paradox can be demonstrated by looking at *base* numerical systems.

Base 10 is most commonly used for daily math applications. We are prone to take *base* 10 as *a given*. It is fairly straight forward and seems inherently logical.

We start with the numbers 1 through 9. To get to the tens column, zero out the one's column and put a 1 in front of the 0, thus getting 10.

Repeat the same procedure to get to the hundreds column as well as any other column.

In grade school, the abstract concept of *base* numerical systems is introduced. Any number can be converted to any different *base* system. Therefore, a *base* 10 number like 974 can be converted to *base* 2, 16 or 20. The number of *base* systems is unlimited.

One way to convert 974 from *base* 10 to *base* 2 is to divide 974 by 2, leaving the remainder as the last number of the *base* 2. Continue this division process until the answer has only zeroes and ones left. The answer is 11 1100 1110.

In *base* 16 the answer is 3CE and in *base* 20 the answer is 28E. *Base* 16 and 20 use the numbers 0 through 9 and then letters to represent the remaining numbers up to 16 and 20 respectively. There are good conversion programs on the internet if you don't want to try and figure out conversions long hand.

I have specifically chosen *base* 2, 16 and 20 due to common functional applications. With the advent of the computer, binary or *base* 2 is the obvious numeric language for programming. Using the least number of variables, 0's and 1's gives us the highest specificity and control, as well as the ability to identify mistakes or problems and make corrections. *Base* 16, which is hexadecimal, is commonly used in web page coding to indicate colors or color proportions. *Base* 20 is the foundation of the *Mayan* numerical system.

Without being able to recognize this and convert back to *base* 10, the *Mayan* calendar would be incomprehensible.

Using the pencil analogy, as an example of paradox: when is a pencil smooth and rough? When is a pencil solid and in material flux? When is a pencil stationary and moving? The answer to all three questions is at the same time. The reason that the answer is true is due to our ability to perceive or conceive the pencil on more than one perceptual level.

Here is a mathematical cross over representation of paradox. When is 974 the same as 11 1100 1110 or 3CE or 28E? The answer is, at the same time.

To our normal linear *mind-brain,* without an awareness or understanding of *base* numerical systems, we would say with confidence and conviction that the above numbers and answers are false and be willing to defend our position against opposition.

Here is a framework and basis, to actively practice and develop the art of *suspension of judgment.*

This, like my definition of *faith,* offers a foundation for contraction and expansion leading to more and more expansion, not clouded by hearsay, bias, unsubstantiated belief, fear of the seemingly unknown or dogma. An authentic window of self-discovery awaits any who would diligently apply the tools and techniques offered in the pages to come. Our natural state is to *be in joy and* have fun.

From the Inside Out

The primary *source* of information from which I frame or define words, terms or phrases in different or unique ways is mainly from an internal *source.* This same internal *source* has led to the development of *RST* and *RMM,* as well as many of the insights and conclusions shared throughout the book. Numerous external source references are also utilized for increased clarity.

Everything I have learned, discovered and share in my writing is not new. I have not invented or created something new with *RST* and *RMM.* Insights or conclusions I share throughout my book that may seem novel or different, or reflect some unique understanding of the nature of our existence or meaning in the universe, are not new either.

My personal experience and awareness has led me to the conclusion that what I am writing and sharing about is a *process* of *awakening and remembering*.

The key term here is *remembering*. I give a personal name or acronym to my therapy.

I share my personal connecting of dots from modern science and spirituality. Whatever I share or frame, in specific ways, is a filtering of data and input through my own spirit, mind and *being*. My perception of what I am writing and sharing is a *remembering of ancient sacred knowledge*. I take no credit for inventing, creating or discovering anything new about our world, our place or purpose in it.

I am humbly grateful to the universe and the divine to be used as a channel or *conduit* to share my own awakening journey and offer others a roadmap they might utilize for themselves.

I offer many pieces of information, perceived, interpreted and utilized. Like the example of a pencil, perceived through multiple levels of perceptual awareness, each level is correct and represents a piece of a more expanded perception and awareness of a whole. There is always a *plus factor*.

We can Remember our Birth

Let's go back, way back, starting at our birth. If you ask most people if they remember their birth, they usually say, *no.* We all have the potential to remember our birth, so why don't we?

Partly this is due to the authoritative control exerted by our family, social, cultural and religious heritage and indoctrination. Most of us are born *tabula rasa* or as a blank slate.

We may believe or conjecture that we existed prior to this birth but generally we don't seem to remember any details.

There is a spiritual mandate for us not to have any memory of the details of our prior existence that is in direct proportion to our ability to consciously remember the transition from life to death and death to life. This is essentially a self-induced projection or acceptance of limitation.

The same external authority that suggests we cannot remember our birth tells us that the answers to the big questions: what am I, where am I, how did I get here, what am I doing here and where am I going, are either not answerable or can only be answered from a religious or scientific framework. Both of these options, although useful, are not adequate.

Religious frameworks often have no individualized personal knowledge or experiential base. They are commonly dependent on an external authority, in the form of books, priests, gurus or others. We must believe or have *blind faith* in them. Science frameworks may seem to have more knowledge or experiential foundations, however, this is primarily true for actual scientists and not the average person. Non-scientists often accept the authority of books and scientists with the same *blind-faith* accepted in religion.

We experience radios, televisions, automobiles and airplanes. Even though some of us may be able to make or fix them, do we truly understand how they work, or do most of us merely accept them as miracles of science? I use the word miracle intentionally, since for many, science is their religion.

Many practicing this new religion of science would deny that it is a religion, however, looking at its practice closely, it resembles a religion in most aspects. Through science, despite the fact that we are able to manipulate forces in nature, as well as manipulate specific things we rarely, if ever, understand the causal mechanisms of how and what we manipulate.

In physics, science is coming closer to a seeming proof of the *Big Bang Theory,* (1). Even if we could or would prove that *space-time* was started from some primordial caldron or hot spot as a *Big Bang*, will that information enhance understanding of our place and purpose in the big picture? Are we approaching a *Unified Field Theory,* (2); a reconciliation between aspects of *Quantum Mechanics,* the extremely small atomic and sub-atomic levels with aspects of *General Relativity,* the extremely large solar systems, galaxies and multi-universe levels?

The blindness of science is its ability to answer technical inquiries or give proofs that side step or ignore fundamental questions.

Even when the *Big Bang* and a *Unified Field Theory* are deemed historical facts from a purely scientific perspective, a definitive answer as to what, where, why or how we exist remains unanswered.

The answer to these fundamental questions would be a *Theory of Everything.*

Religion does a much better job with these fundamental questions, however, in most of its forms offers little or no tools for personal experiential proof.

Here is a tool box filled with resources for the individual to find their own unique *Theory of Everything* from an experiential framework. This process reconciles both religion and science, two parts of a much greater whole. In the movie *Thor* the character Thor says, *I come from a world in which science and magic are one and the same.* I agree, as this is true for me as well.

Besides the accepted mandate that we can't remember our birth, for most of us, the birth experience has a traumatic component. One of the tools we use as a survival or coping mechanism is to suppress or block the memory of traumatic events.

In a normal birth, as we are being pushed out of the birth canal, we start to experience waves of pressure against our body. These waves are intense and often framed as uncomfortable.

Our subconscious remembers this experience and starts to project a pattern of avoidance, like bracing against the front of a roller coaster and realizing that there is no turning back, feeling both exhilarated and scared. The pressure continues to build and build, primarily on the head. Our anxiety is increasing. All of a sudden there is a pop! Where are we? The air is too cold. The boundary between our body and the new external environment is unclear.

Sounds are too intense, light is too bright. Our attempt to cry out, to connect, is ineffective. We may be in shock or panic at this point. Often we receive a slap on our backside that sends waves of increased sensations throughout our body and our panic grows.

As we start to remember this experience, is it any wonder that we have deeply suppressed it. The trauma is too intense. We can't risk holding this memory as it may interfere with or limit any further development.

This is a curious paradox. The memory of our birth is an important developmental link. It is our connection of the memory as a trauma, having both a negative physical and emotional component that induces our self-activated *avoidance* and *disconnect* mechanism.

This mechanism is under our *free will* and self-control. Due to its extremely rapid activation, we may perceive it or frame it as an unconscious reflex. A seemingly unconscious reflex is derived from a prior conscious awareness or experience.

Our ability to frame a response as unconscious allows us to support a perception that some responses are not in our control. This is a self-perpetuating negative feedback loop that is just another suppressed memory.

As a seeming survival mechanism, we block the memory, the memory that is still intact when we start to open our hearts to the moment and move into *unconditionalness*.

To be *unconditional* is to choose to not place a condition or judgment on our memories, experiences, wishes, projections, persons, places or things. This *unconditional* choice is to resist the temptation to frame anything as good or bad, right or wrong.

As we are held and pressed to the chest, thump thump... thump thump. We experience the rhythm the beat of life, the *in-flow and out-flow*. We remember the ocean, the womb, the fluid, the warmth, the security. *Oh my! I'm not there, where am I, where am I?* The panic mounts again. We desperately try to orient. As we develop, we are drawn to spontaneously place our hand or another body part in our mouth, pressing our jaw against it, increasing our sensation of pressure. This pressure causes us to pull our hand away in a jerk. We see a shadow move in front of our face and are unable to focus. We discover our hand in our mouth again, now our foot, over and over until *déjà vu* (3) occurs. *I am a body*!

Through proprioceptive; sensory feedback, we discover and verify. Yes we are a body, our first science experiment is a rousing success. Wait, we are not a body; the body is only a shell.

We are not the body; the body is only a shell? If we are not the body, then what are we? Clearly it seems from all the external evidence that of course we are a body. Who are you trying to fool, yes *we are bodies*!

The body is energy; physically it is mostly empty space yet fragile and perishable. Energy can be transmuted but not destroyed. It moves from one state to another. We are energy. We are consciousness. We are a unit of consciousness.

Our ability to confirm that we are a body, as well as our ability to consciously transcend the body, is dependent on our awareness of the fascial membrane.

What is the *Fascia*?

Fascia is a transparent membrane, thinner than tissue paper that surrounds every muscle. Looking at a cross section of muscle magnified, it is made up of bundles of fibers with each bundle being surrounded by a fascial sheath. *Fascia* surrounds and intimately interlaces throughout all body tissues and structures. Continuing this visual journey at the ends of muscles, the ligaments are also surrounded by *fascia*, which attaches to the bones as the periosteum. *Fascia* surrounds every joint, nerve, blood vessel and lymphatic duct. *Fascia* crosses the blood brain barrier, encasing all the meninges, as well as every brain structure. *Fascia* surrounds every organ. The heart has the pericardial sac, the lungs the pleural sac.

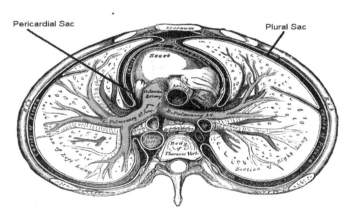

Fig. 2

PLEURAL and PERICARDIAL SACS:

(black inner ring lining)

The diaphragm is a special thickened membrane of *fascia* that separates the upper and lower abdominal organs. The eardrum is the thickest layer of body *fascia*.

It is transparent and, other than the eye, is the only part of *fascia* in direct contact with the external world. This direct contact gives the tympanic membrane which is the eardrum a special and unique function in relation to body calibration. Proper body calibration is crucial for increasing our range for both transmission and reception of signals. These signals extend well beyond the range of our limited five component sensory apparatus.

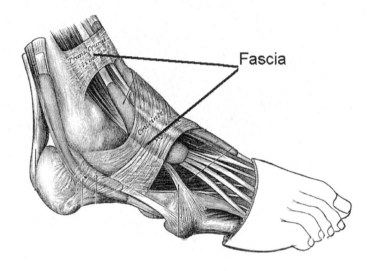

Fascia

Fig. 3

FASCIA of FOOT

Fascia is Everywhere

Fascia is the only part of the human body that is 100% *contiguous,* or connected everywhere. It is an exceptionally important part of our bodies. This structure is an organ, as well as a membrane. Skin is referred to as an organ. It has been suggested that it is the largest organ of the body. *Fascia* is by many factors or multiples significantly larger than the skin.

There is a shifting paradigm placing an emphasis on the importance and function of membranes. In Bruce Lipton's book, *The Biology of Belief*,(4) he shares the observation that when you remove the nucleus of a cell, it will still function, while if you remove the membrane of the cell it collapses and dies.

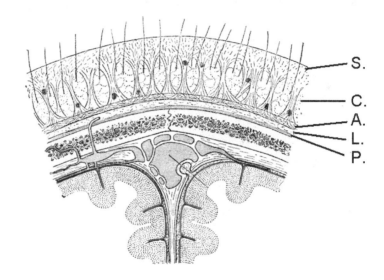

Fig. 4

FIVE LAYERS of HUMAN SCALP: Demonstrates Complexity of Fascial Membrane; S=skin, C=connective tissue, A=aponeurosis, L=loose areolar connective tissue, P=the pericranium as the periosteum.

String Theory

In physics, a theoretical cosmologic idea known as *String Theory*, (5) suggests that everything is made up of vibrating strings of sub-atomic proportions coming together to form membranes called *Branes*.

The term *Brane* might be transposed as *Brain* since it is the membrane that controls and defines the shape and function of everything.

With an individual cell, the membrane, not the nucleus, determines survivability. The historical concept equating the nucleus as the brain of the cell is being superseded by the new paradigm of the cell membrane as the brain of the cell. The concept of membranes as having quintessential properties is being recognized from the sub-atomic level to that of galaxies and everything in between, including inter-dimensional space.

The vibrational quality or frequency of the strings is the *cause substrate* that defines the character or shape of the strings into a membrane. Once the membrane forms, the energy matrix, or *Chi,* can fill the membrane to manifest as a thing. In *String Theory*, larger *Branes* of differing vibrational sound frequencies establish a series of dimensions. There are many differing mathematical constructs or individual string theories. The development of *M Theory* has successfully integrated all the differing string theories into one. *M Theory*, (6) postulates the presence of eleven dimensions.

In *M Theory*, the premise that there are eleven dimensions mandates eleven primary energy membranes with different frequency and vibrational states.

These frequencies extend beyond the range of scientific equipment to verify. Their existence is non-physical and based on purely theoretical or mathematical extrapolations. Within each of these eleven primary energy membranes, many non-physical things are formed by coalescing membranes that are then filled by the energy matrix.

An experiential framework, outside the confines of the mind and linear thought, can prove on an individual basis the reality of different dimensions of differing vibrational frequencies.

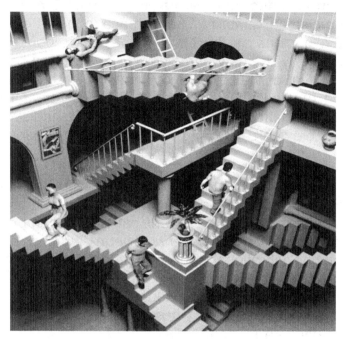

Fig. 5

IMAGE RESEMBLING MC ESCHER'S (RELAVITY)

(This image demonstrates graphically the perception of multiple dimensions as expressed by *String Theory*).

Fascia=Membranes=Compartments=

Structures=Organs

Observing a human egg; it is a mass of genetic material that is encased in a membrane. Without this membrane, the possibility of fertilization, leading to cell division, and the continuing growth of a fetus is nil.

Once the egg is fertilized, follow the image as it divides in half, then quarters, to eventually become its complete manifest *form*.

It is the presence of more and more membranes forming an increased number of compartments that allows complexity and differentiation into different organs and structures. These membranes are the early web of *fascia* also present in a fully developed adult.

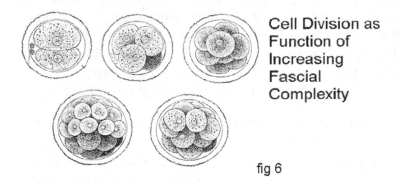

Cell Division as Function of Increasing Fascial Complexity

fig 6

DIVIDING HUMAN EGG

Sound Creates Vibration

In *String Theory*, the vibration of the strings is conjectured to have a musical quality. Is it sound that induces vibration or vibration that induces sound? In the physical universe, the evidence is that vibration, as in the plucking of a guitar string, makes the sound. The sound wave emanating from a tuning fork that has been struck causes a second stationary tuning fork, of the same note, to vibrate and make sound.

The sound wave produced from the primary tuning fork induces the second tuning fork to vibrate and make sound as a consequence of the principles of *harmonics* and *resonance* in action. The question of sound or vibration, as primary, must be held in the same non-logical, non-linear perspective as the *Chicken or the Egg Paradox,* as to which came first.

Vibration within *space-time* is a physical phenomenon, bound by physical laws. Sound, although physical, extends through a frequency band-width that is also non-physical and crosses the last membrane that defines the border of *STEM;* s*pace-time,* energy and matter. This is my use of the acronym *STEM* as differentiated from the common educational application where STEM stands for; science, technology, engineering and math.

In *String Theory* sound creates differing vibrating frequency patterns. These coalesce to *form* strings; pulsating units of differing sound-vibrational frequencies, which continue to coalesce to *form* membranes. Membranes define the edge or energetic *blue-print* that *source* fills with spirit *Chi* to *form* different dimensions, or different objects, both physical and non-physical.

Genes

At the physical level, genes are part of the physical manifestation of the energetic matrix. Neither the nucleus in an individual cell nor the genes exclusively control, regulate or determine the *form* nor function of a cell, organ, system or person. Membranes, from the sub-atomic to the macrocosmic level, play a critical, yet to be fully recognized, understood or utilized role relative to all *form* and function.

Sound is the Key

The most common form of yoga is *Hatha Yoga*. (7) This is a system of physical postures and breathing techniques to improve health and expand awareness through unwinding and release of *fascia*. There are twelve primary systems of yoga. One of the twelve is *Shabda Yoga* (8), the yoga of the Sound Current. In this system of yoga it is recognized that the sound or, *shab*, is the creating and sustaining force of existence. Through the use of *mantra* or sound chanting, a body harmonic can be induced that causes *resonance* with the *shab* or living word. As we induce this *resonance*, it allows our consciousness to enter into a larger, broader awareness inherent in this wave *form*. This *process* is augmented as we surrender with trust and abandon to the *mantra*.

Mantra

A well-known mantra is *Aum* or *Om*. This simple syllable, when chanted with an *unconditional* open heart, can catalyze meaningful change. To the mind, this may seem ludicrous or even nonsensical.

How can a verbal sound have that kind of power? Intellectual conjecture will never bring anyone closer to solving this question. Implementing this mantra with discipline and commitment can demonstrate whether it has any true value or merit. Its use does not require a belief system to function. Its mode of action is consistently reproducible and teachable.

In the Beginning was the Word

In the Christian Bible from John1:1, *In the beginning was the word, and the word was with God and the word was God.*(9) In *Shabda Yoga,* the word is pure sound and an audible living force. This sound is spirit, the same spirit identified in all religions and a synonym for *Chi.* This spirit force has a dual aspect of sound and light. Sound is the creative force and light is its reflection through *space-time.*

Cymatics

In the study of vibratory actinics, more commonly known as *cymatics*, it can be demonstrated how sound causes particles of sand to take on different geometric shapes like triangles or hexagrams.

Wikipedia states, *Cymatics is the study of wave phenomena. It is typically associated with the physical patterns produced through the interaction of sound waves in a medium. A simple experiment demonstrating the visualization of cymatics can be done by sprinkling sand on a metal plate and vibrating the plate, for example by drawing a violin bow along the edge, the sand will then form itself into standing wave patterns such as simple concentric circles.*

The higher the frequency, the more complex the shapes produced, with certain shapes having similarities to traditional mandala designs. (10)

A Mandala is a circle with simple to complex geometric shapes inside that demonstrate symmetry or organization. The edge that is the boundary of the circle represents a membrane. The complexity of geometric shapes within the circle is induced as a function of increasing membranes.

Gregg Braden-Awakening to Zero Point

In Gregg Braden's video series, *Awakening to Zero Point*, (11) he shows an example of *cymatics* using plant spores of mugwort which is (lycopodium). Changing the sound, stagnant geometric forms become moving vortices that resemble miniature stellar spiral nebulae.

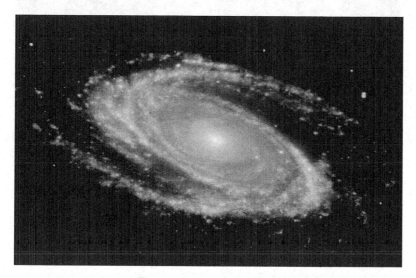

Fig 7

SPIRAL NEBULA

As-Above - So-Below

This shape is not coincidental, it is a reflection of the *process* of creation and an acknowledgement of the spiritual principle, *as-above - so-below*. This is the *macrocosm* and *microcosm*, being reflections of each other. To see *cymatic* images, do a web search or look up Dr. Hans Jenny, the Father of *Cymatics*. (12)

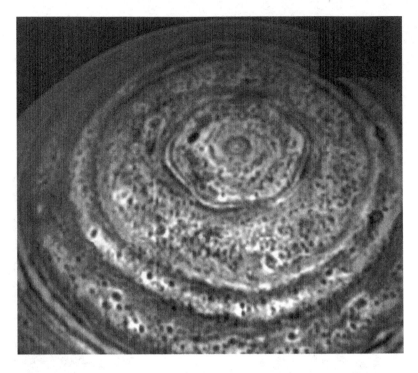

Fig. 8

NORTH POLAR HEXAGONAL, CYMATIC,
CLOUD Feature on Saturn, discovered by
Voyager and confirmed in 2006 by Cassini

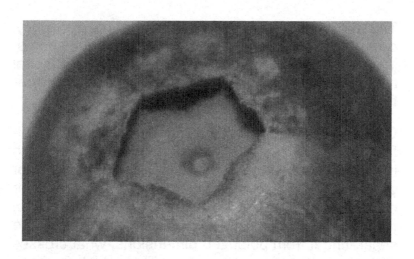

Fig. 9

PENTAGONAL POLYGON: Top of Blueberry

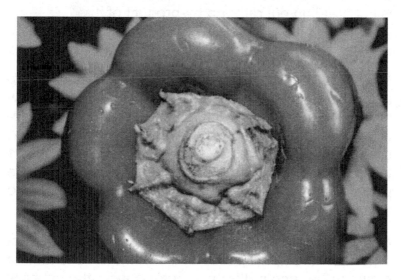

Fig.10

HEXAGONAL POLYGON: Top of Bell Pepper

The spiral nebulae shape induced by sound, frequency, *cymatic* manipulation of mugwort (lycopodium) spores, is a micro reflection of full sized macro-cosmic spiral nebulae. The blueberry and bell pepper are micro reflections of the *Hexagon on Saturn*.

Creation emanates from the domain of the un-manifest, non-polarized, no-thing dimensions. That which is created and creates, exists outside the borders or domain of *STEM; space-time*, energy and matter. The created has no beginning or end, it has neither *form* nor density. Creation does not cross the membrane separating it from polarized dimensions, what crosses is the manifestation of creation. That which is manifest takes on all the properties and characteristics of *STEM*. Qualities of the manifest include *form* and varying degrees of mass or density. That which has mass is a manifestation of the creative *process*. Manifestation is not creation but rather a by-product of it.

Powers of Ten

Powers of Ten, is a short film. (13) It starts with an image of a couple on a beach. The camera scene now pulls away from the beach. Each new scene is an increase of magnification by a factor of ten. The next scene, as the camera moves up into the sky, first shows the coastline, than the North American continent, the planet Earth, our solar system, other star systems and galaxies beyond.

A striking aspect of these magnified images, is the vast distances of empty space, as the camera continues to move further and further into outer-space; the physical space of our universe moving away from the couple on the beach.

The camera zooms back to the couple on the beach at an accelerated rate. Now the camera reverses the process. Starting from the surface of the skin, each new image is magnified, by the same tenfold factor. An equal number of magnified images, as seen moving out through outer-space, is now seen moving in through deeper and deeper layers of skin, through all body structures, progressing to the sub-atomic particles of inner-space and beyond. The *microcosm* and the *macrocosm* as reflections of each other demonstrate: *As-above - so-below* and *as-within - so-without.*

Chaos as a Higher Order of Perception

Chaos, is a term used to define something that our mind is incapable of perceiving in a linear fashion. What the mind cannot organize or systematize, it will categorize as part of, or being derived from *chaos*. This abstract concept defines a place, space or thought as being devoid of any recognizable pattern, organization or *form*. *Chaos* is defined by what it is not, rather than by what it is. This is a unique property of *chaos*, a crude way to attempt defining the undefinable. The *mind-brain* can only approach *chaos* from a linear, limited perspective.

When mental perception is blocked or inaccessible, an actual doorway or access point of *transcendent* awareness exists. *Chaos* is a more expanded order of perception or consciousness that cannot be accessed through the mind or simple linear cognition, it is *transcendent*. That which is *transcendent* does not originate from the *mind-brain*. It comes from *Source.*

It comes from a higher order of intelligence or consciousness, emanating from the *no-thing* realm. This book is a primer to find and activate this guiding energy.

A physical membrane is a sound, energy, vibrational abstract made manifest. In the human body this manifests as the fascial membrane. This fascial membrane is the barrier that defines the transition from *chaos* to organization, from the un-manifest to the manifest. That which creates and crosses this membrane and functions as the carrier wave for consciousness, is consciousness itself. This consciousness expresses itself as the creative force, spirit, voice of God, word, logos, sound or *shab*. Once consciousness enters the physical body it is *fascia* that it travels on and in. *Fascia is the seat of consciousness.* The brain is just more densely wound layers of *fascia*. Consciousness is neither limited nor bound by the brain.

The physical fascial membrane surrounding all parts of the body is a multiple layered sac. It is the same membrane that is the template matrices forming all sub-atomic particles, as well as the membrane encapsulating the first complete cell. It is the membrane in the fertilized egg that splits the egg into two, four, eight, sixteen and all consecutive compartments. These compartments are the template matrices for all body parts and organs.

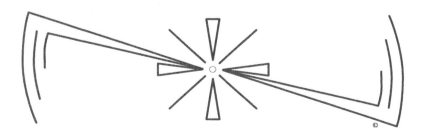

As we wake up and consciously connect with body *fascia*, we take back control of every organ, system and function of the body. The physical *fascia* of our body is connected to *fascia* of the Earth. Qualities characteristic of *fascia* are universal. Earth *fascia,* like body *fascia*, is the carrier membrane of consciousness. Our living Earth mother, *Gaia*, utilizes her *fascia* just like us. Her *fascia* is connected to the *fascia* of the solar system, galaxy and universe. The difference between these fascial layers or membranes called *Branes* from *String Theory*, as well as all fascial membranes, both manifest and un-manifest is their differentiation of sound, energy, vibrational, frequency states.

RST and *RMM* are tools to help us maintain health, *well-being* and energetic equilibrium, by connecting to and un-winding *fascia*. They are also a medium for connecting with all levels of existence. From the micro to macro-cosmic physical dimensions, as well as all non-physical dimensions, they are tools to link us through *fascia* to personal experience and the discovery of our place, purpose and meaning.

Our ability to engage an intellectual dialogue about the validity or accuracy of the purpose of body *fascia*, or further extrapolations about membranes, or the significance of sound in relationship to creation as manifestation, is mental hyperbole. This type of mental abstraction will not increase our potential for understanding, or awareness, nor will it catalyze a direct experience that is *transcendent*. William James (14) used the term *Numinosity*, popularized by Rudolf Otto, (15) to identify a *transcendent* state of spiritual *being*, a space connected to and guided by divine presence.

Robert Heinlein-*Grock*

Grock is a term coined by Robert Heinlein in his book *Stranger in a Strange Land.*(16) To *grock* is to *be* in a state in which we enter into a type of symbiotic relationship with *it*; where *it* is anything, whether physical or non-physical, where the borders of self and non-self blur and we become *that* which we perceive. As we *Grock, it,* we experience an awareness of *oneness.*

A stage in our journey of spiritual awakening or enlightenment is an experiential state where the perceptual border of self and non-self is absent. This state generates a personal awareness of the connectedness of everyone and everything. In this state, the statement, we are one, is not derived from a mental process or any external scientific authority. To *grock* a single thing is a developmental step on the journey to *grock* everything.

Numinosity is an essential component of this *process. RST* and *RMM* are powerful tools to catalyze the *Numinous* to help us wake up and remember our divine birth-right, to *grock* it all. The experiential link into the *oneness* is not the end point or final destination, it is the beginning of a seemingly new, yet ancient door way; *A Journey for Personal Self-Discovery, Awakening, and Healing.*

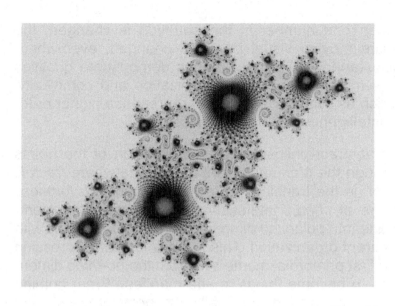

Fig. 11

FRACTAL IMAGE

Dr. Mandelbrot and *Fractals*

Dr. Benoit B. Mandelbrot (17) is a mathematician who developed an equation using binomials: $z_{n+1} = z_n^2 + c$, where c and z are complex numbers and n is zero or a positive integer or natural number. This equation when run as a computer program makes *fractal* images. The first visual extrapolation of this formula is called the *Mandelbrot Set*, shown in figure 12. The set is made up of circular shapes. Shapes have edges; the intersection of these edges *form* membranes. The equation is a symbolic representation forming complex *fractal* images through the edge membrane of the *Mandelbrot Set*. These *fractals* are of unlimited variety and complexity.

When one number in the equation is changed, the entire moving visual *fractal* is changed, everywhere simultaneously. *Fractal* images demonstrate qualities of symmetry, repetition, organization and complexity, which as symbols, suggest or represent a higher order of intelligence or consciousness.

An abstract philosophical interpretation of the points through the *Mandelbrot Set* membrane where *fractals form*, is the transition from the *un-manifest*, *formless* realm of *chaos*, intersecting and crossing the membrane into polarized dimensions to manifest *forms* with inherent organization. This is the *un-manifest* crossing the first primordial membrane from the *no-thing* dimension to become things, made manifest. From nothing comes everything, poetically, the point of creation or more accurately the point of manifestation.

Fractals

The direction and flow of the forming *fractals* is from the inside moving out. This is an important observation that portents the significance of change as being generated from an internal *process*. Change can be catalyzed from the outside, but change itself is a function of *out-flow*. This topic is addressed in more detail in a later section of the book.

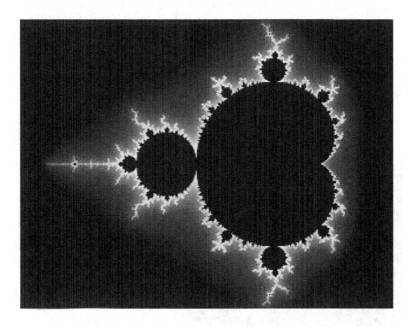

Fig. 12

MANDELBROT SET

From Wikipedia; *Image gallery of a zoom sequence.
The Mandelbrot set shows more intricate detail the
closer one looks or magnifies the image, usually called
"zooming in". The following example of an image sequence zooming to a selected c value gives an im-
pression of the infinite richness of different geometri-
cal structures, and explains some of their typical rules.
The magnification of the last image relative to the first
one is about 10,000,000,000(B) to 1. Relating to an or-
dinary (computer) monitor, it represents a section of a
Mandelbrot set with a diameter of 4 million kilometers.
Its border would show an inconceivable number of different fractal structures.*

MULTIPLE PROGRESSIVE *FRACTAL* IMAGES, Figs. 13-26

The large box shows the magnification from the image above it, marked by the small inner box.

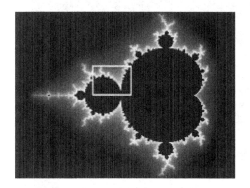

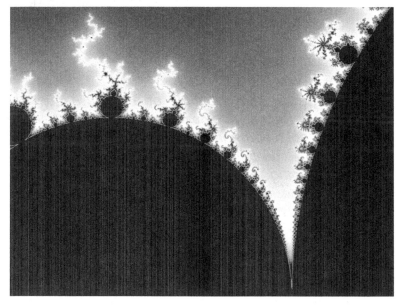

Fig.13

The large box shows the magnification from the image above it, marked by the small inner box.

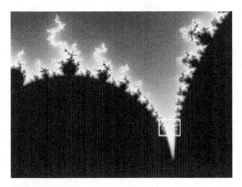

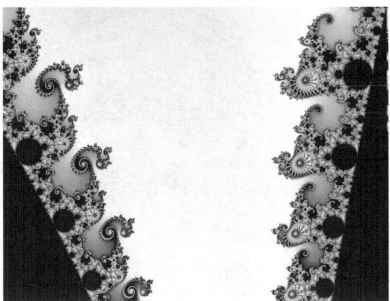

Fig. 14

The large box shows the magnification from the image above it, marked by the small inner box.

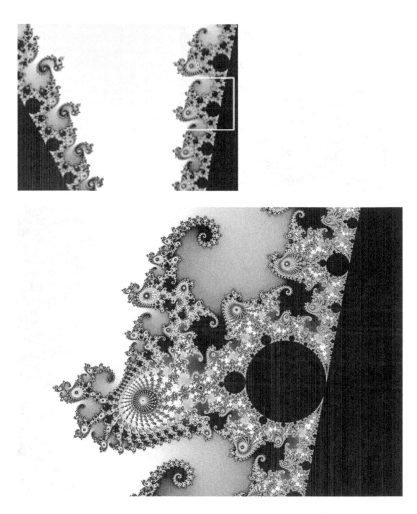

Fig. 15

The large box shows the magnification from the
image above it, marked by the small inner box.

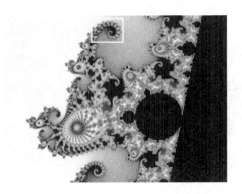

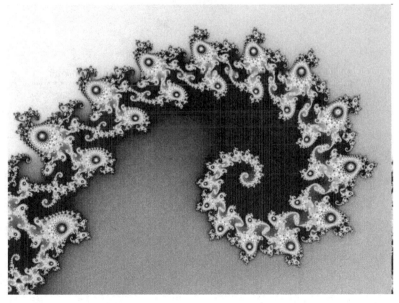

Fig. 16

The large box shows the magnification from the
image above it, marked by the small inner box.

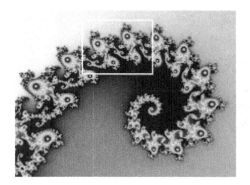

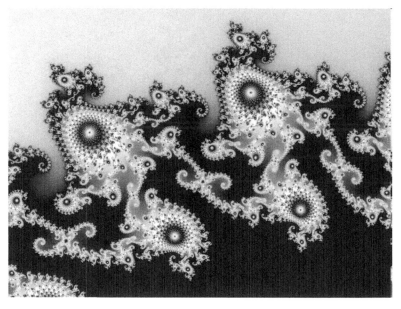

Fig. 17

The large box shows the magnification from the image above it, marked by the small inner box.

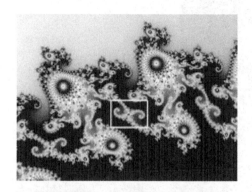

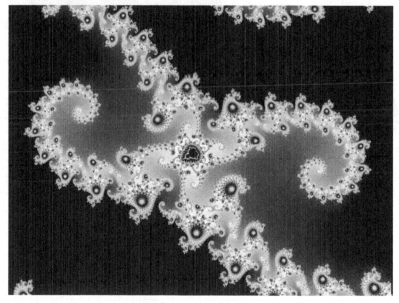

Fig. 18

The large box shows the magnification from the image above it, marked by the small inner box.

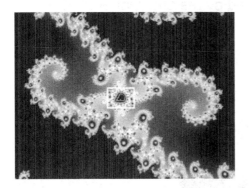

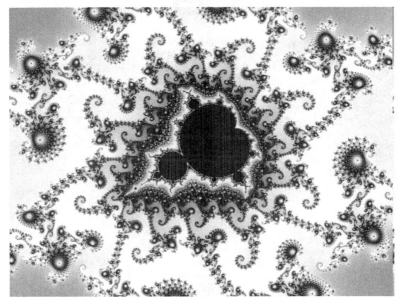

Fig. 19

The large box shows the magnification from the
image above it, marked by the small inner box.

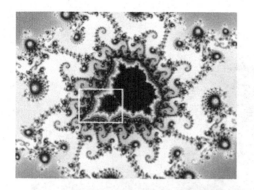

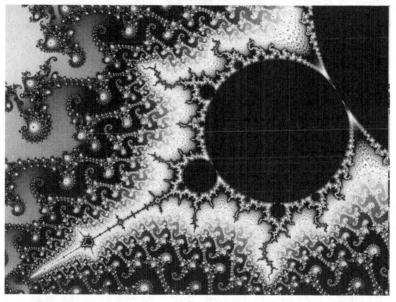

Fig. 20

The large box shows the magnification from the image above it, marked by the small inner box.

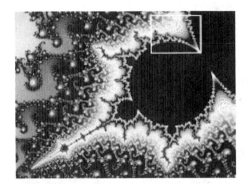

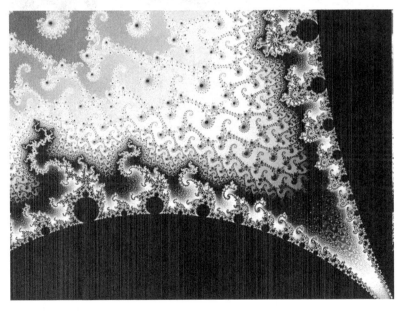

Fig. 21

The large box shows the magnification from the
image above it, marked by the small inner box.

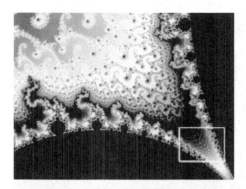

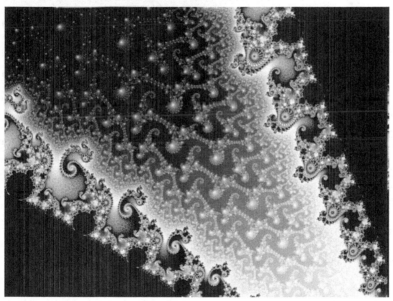

Fig. 22

The large box shows the magnification from the image above it, marked by the small inner box.

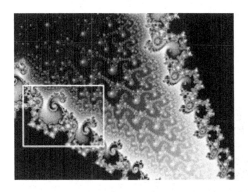

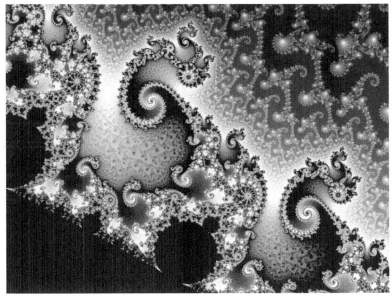

Fig. 23

The large box shows the magnification from the image above it, marked by the small inner box.

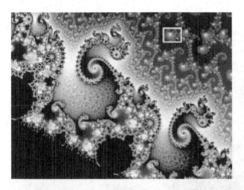

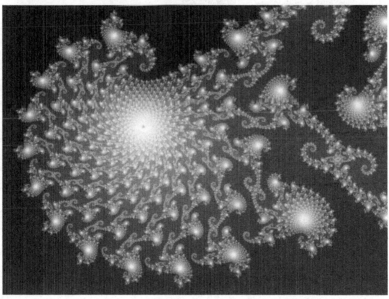

Fig. 24

The large box shows the magnification from the image above it, marked by the small inner box.

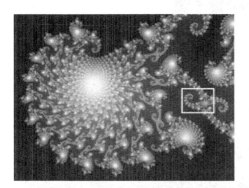

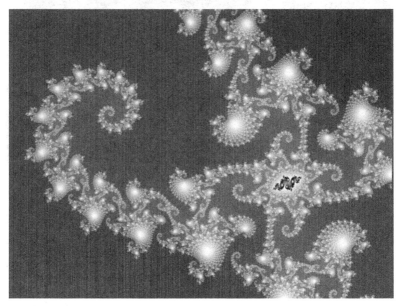

Fig. 25

The large box shows the magnification from the image above it, marked by the small inner box.

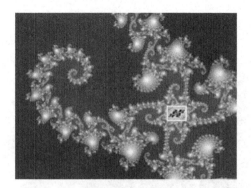

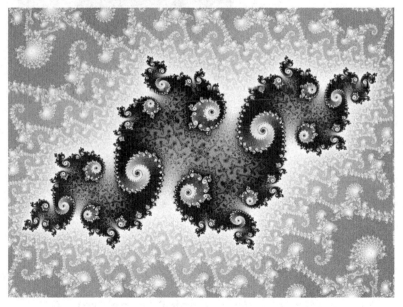

Fig. 26

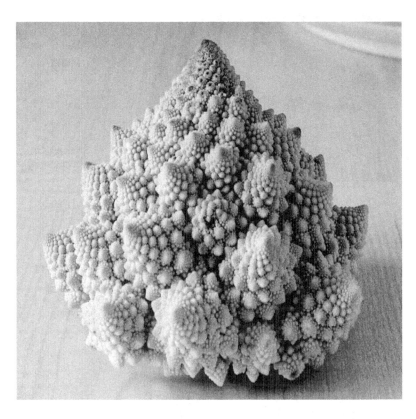

Fig. 27

ROMANESCO BROCCOLI

(Showing *fractal*, spirals in nature)

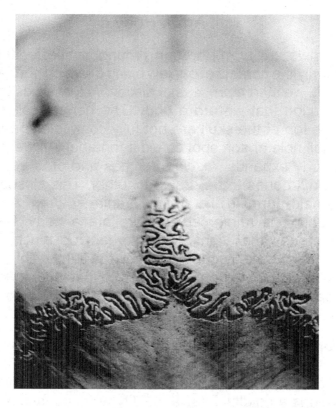

Fig. 28

SUTURES (FROM DEER SKULL)
AS *FRACTALS*

Through proprioceptive feedback; the feedback loop between the central and peripheral nervous systems, we increase fascial twisting, pulling the sutures of the skull bones together. The sutures of the skull bones are *fractal* patterns. They are a physical manifestation of the *Mandelbrot Set* and represent the interface between the manifest; the body, and the *un-manifest*, pure consciousness that is not bound by a body.

I Am a Body

When we are born, through proprioceptive feedback; primarily the contact of our jaw biting down on our hands or feet, we start a *process* of discovery that leads to the realization that we are a body. The bones that make up the top of the skull are not fully connected, leaving a small hole or soft spot called a fontanel. As we grow, the body expands, *fascia* stretches and pulls causing the skull bones to be drawn together. This closes the fontanels, forming the *fractal* cranial sutures. As our perception is reinforced that we are a body, fascial membranes may tighten and torque too much. This may pull the skull bones together, too tightly. This is an all too common dis-equilibrium state that increases the probability of our essence or consciousness becoming sealed into the body shell.

When our consciousness is sealed into the physical shell of our body it limits our ability to access or utilize any *transcendent* input. As *fascia* winds excessively it develops a rigidity. Fascial rigidity reduces fascial permeability. With reduced permeability, the normal, natural, completely unrestricted flow of life force, as *Chi,* is compromised. Reduction in life force causes imbalances leading to symptoms and diseases. Total permeability is the natural state of the membrane and is a critical factor in health maintenance and expanding consciousness.

At birth, the top of the head, from a superior view; from the top down, has a hole anterior; toward the front, called the frontal fontanel. This is the largest hole in a developing skull and corresponds to the crown *chakra*.

The *chakras* are energy vortices that have correspondences and influence control over endocrinologic organs. More on this topic will follow, further in the book. The crown *chakra*, has been suggested from many divergent spiritual sources, as the most common site where consciousness enters the body at birth. If these *fractal* sutures; the jagged edged interface of the skull bones, seal too firmly, normal expansion and contraction of the skull, as well as the rest of the body, is restricted.

One consequence of this sutural jamming is the potential to become a permanent resident in the body. Isn't being what you call a resident in the body, not only normal and natural but essential and not a topic of debate or conjecture? This type of total identification, without any hesitation or question of self as inexorably linked to a body, is a testament to the effectiveness of our familial, social, cultural, educational indoctrination to limit and narrow our view or perception of self. Having consciousness frozen in the shell that is the physical body for a life-time is neither normal, natural nor healthy. This condition will last until the death of the physical shell unless active steps are taken to reverse it. The implementation of *RST* and *RMM* can facilitate this *process*.

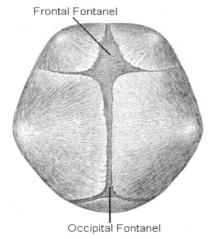

Frontal Fontanel

Occipital Fontanel

From a superior view, at the back of the skull is the posterior (occipital) fontanel. From a lateral or side view is the anterolateral (sphenoidal) fontanel and the posterolateral (mastoid) fontanel.

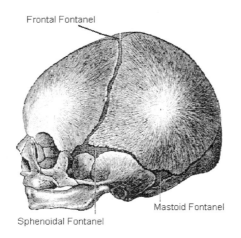

Frontal Fontanel

Mastoid Fontanel

Sphenoidal Fontanel

Fig. 29

INFANT SKULL, OPEN SUTURES(FONTANELS)

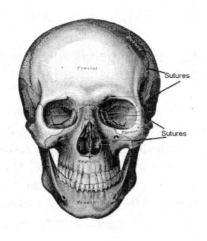

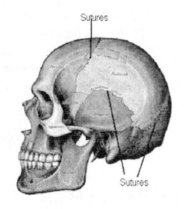

Fig. 30

ADULT SKULL with CLOSED SUTURES

I Am Not a Body

At birth, while the fascial membrane remains permeable, we move our consciousness freely in and out of the body from any *chakra*. Babies remain on a cusp for a variable time interval deciding whether to commit to a body shell. The body is to be utilized and understood as a transitional state in our personal journey of self-discovery and awakening. The interval for body commitment of a newly born child, is determined by how rapidly it embraces and fixates on the parameters of its self-perceived, projected *be-mi;* body, ego, mind and identity.

It is normal and natural that consciousness chooses a body *form*. It is not natural that consciousness fixate or be limited to a body *form*. If this fixation is actualized, we must recognize and reverse the *process* of solidification, if we are to function as *cause* rather than *effect*. Our birth-right is to learn to use a body, to have experiences and expand awareness and ultimately, to be freed through conscious intent and action from the body, rather than be bound by it. Until this freedom is accomplished, we will remain the *effect* of our own causation.

The challenge that the universe, or the divine, offers is to achieve freedom of consciousness from the body shell, in this specific life. If this freedom is not actualized in this life, the risk is being caught in a self-perpetuating negative feed-back loop of repeating experience binding us to the body until the cycle can be broken permanently.

The Body is Just a Shell-I Am *Soul*

What is the fascial membrane permeable to, and what is the value to us? The membrane is permeable to two things. First, it is permeable to consciousness. If the body is just a shell and we are not the body, then what are we? We are a unit of consciousness or particle of awareness called *soul*. We are *soul*, we have a body. We are not a body that has a *soul*. This is a critical and important differentiation. The body is impermanent and perishable, *soul* is eternal.

Secondly, the fascial membrane is permeable to *Chi*. *Chi* is an energy *form*, synonymous with spirit. It is a living force coursing through the acupuncture meridians and *chakras*. Food, water and air sustain life proportionally to the amount of *Chi* or life force energy extractable from them. Protein, fat, vitamins, minerals and enzymes in food are not what nourish us. They are physical dimension shells that act as holding repositories for *Chi*. They represent an indirect source of energy.

Understanding and actively being able to utilize this principle allows us to have a very different relationship with air, water and food. This principle potentially changes the premise that there are critical nutrients in specific foods that must be ingested in specific quantities, to maintain life or health. It may be that these dietary mandates, derived from our current knowledge of biochemistry and clinical nutrition, are only accurate and applicable within the domain of a limited spectrum of consciousness.

Throughout history, different spiritual traditions have alluded to individuals that consume little or no physical food, deriving life force energy from more direct sources. In modern times, a variety of Eastern mystical savants have demonstrated to the scientific community varying degrees of this capacity, to live and survive on less and less physical food. One such Indian guru, who was my patient, lived almost exclusively as a fruitarian. He was well into his nineties and seemed able to transmute fruit into whatever his body needed, which he had been doing for decades. The average human, functioning from the limited paradigm or construct of a Western scientific perspective, would die of malnutrition trying to follow such a diet. Did this guru know or understand something that most people choose to frame or believe as fanciful fiction?

Chi, or spirit, has the dual qualities of light and sound. *Chi* is derived from air, water and food, it is also derived from alternate sources. *Chi* can be accessed and channeled utilizing meditation, contemplation, chanting, rhythmic motion, or any combination of these together. *Chi* passes through us. Whether derived from air, water, food or directly, as pure spirit, its nutrient or sustaining properties are released or extracted as it passes through us. This is an important spiritual principle. We can try to hold it exclusively for ourselves and not let it pass through. This is one way we create imbalances that lead to health problems.

Chi access through the body is potentiated when *grounded*. *Grounding* is when the body is in contact with the Earth. *Chi's* effect on physical, emotional, mental and spiritual existence is as the *source* for nourishment, healing, longevity and enlightenment.

Soul is consciousness and spirit is energy. Science and spirituality are not mutually exclusive. With the right understanding, awareness and application they can be brought into concordance.

Grounding

A personal commitment to actively *ground* the body daily is an essential part of health, longevity and spiritual awakening. *Grounding* is necessary to establish and maintain our essential connection with the energy field of the planet. During this *process* body *fascia* and Earth *fascia* are linked. This is done barefoot, standing on dirt, sand, grass, gravel, soil or rock. A slightly reduced connection can be established standing inside on wood, tiles made from ceramic, marble, brick or slate. One-hundred percent wool carpet or rugs increase the field. Laminate flooring, as long as the primary material occurs in nature, is adequate.

For any of these natural materials to be adequately *grounded,* part of their edge must reach the edge of the building foundation. This allows the planet's energy field to arc from the Earth over the concrete slab onto a natural floor. A simple concrete slab, painted or not, has a substantial dampening effect. This is due to its increased physical density and composition.

Synthetic blend carpets or other completely synthetic materials block the Earth's field even more. Synthetic socks should not be used. Cotton or wool or a cotton, wool blend sock is best.

Wearing a one-hundred percent leather moccasin, is excellent. Until the leather of a moccasin is worn in, Earth *Chi* is blocked. *Fascia* embedded in the dead skin (leather) of an animal holds the negative emotional charge of fear and the trauma of the animal's death. As a new moccasin is worn, walking on the Earth, the rotational compression action and natural sounds emulate an *RST* treatment. As *fascia* of the leather unwinds, Earth *Chi* is now able to flow without restriction.

Moccasins are better worn barefoot, however, socks may be used. Footwear made from any natural materials work as well.

Grounding is also accomplished anytime we place our hands, any body part, or our whole body in running water. As long as this running water is coming through a piping system that travels through the ground, the water is *grounded.* Even when the piping system is plastic, as long as the waters source is *grounded* the water retains and carries Earth *Chi.* The Earth *Chi* charge may be diminished but it is still present. Taking a shower, even in a high-rise hotel room, is utilizing *grounded* water.

How long, on a daily basis, is it necessary to be *grounded* to maintain optimal health? Any time interval of *grounding* is useful and significant, from a few minutes to a half an hour or more.

Not long ago every human on this planet was *grounded* 24/7. This is our natural state. It is only in very recent history that we have developed footwear and living surfaces that dis-connect us from the Earth's field. How severe is this problem? The book; *Earthing* by Clinton Ober, Dr. Steven Sinatra and Martin Zucker attempts to answer some of these questions.

Ober describes and explains the field of energy emanating from the surface of planet Earth as electric. All of his recommendations and products are based on the transmission and conduction of this electric field.

The electric portion of Earth's field is the energy that our current technology can readily identify and quantify. The energy or field emanating from the Earth as *Chi,* or life force, expresses itself as a much wider bandwidth than electricity.

Connecting our bodies to the full field of Earth's *Chi,* or life force, I call *grounding.* Current technologies to identify and quantify the full qualities and parameters of *Chi* are inadequate. Limiting the research in *Earthing* technology and recommendations to the electric field is a logical step, as it has the highest capacity for scientific credibility and reproducibility at this time.

How important is the electric portion of Earth's *Chi* field relative to the field as a whole? The answer to this question is currently unknown. The axiom derived from natural medicine that *the whole is greater than the sum of its parts* is a good starting reference point to pursue more definitive answers and guidance.

Another aspect of *grounding* involves a mechanism to potentiate the *Chi* field force passing through our bodies from the Earth. Connecting to the Earth, through a *grounded* interface is no longer sufficient, by itself, to protect us from disease, or to ensure or generate optimal health.

There may have been an historic time when the Earth was less polluted and life was simpler that *grounding* alone may have been enough. Today, because of planetary ionizing radiation, radioactive isotopes, xenobiotics like synthetic chemicals, solvents , drugs, petroleum by-products, plastics, pesticides, herbicides, genetically modified plants and animals, radio waves, x-rays, micro-waves and a seemingly endless list of toxins, our bodies and psyches balancing, compensatory mechanisms are overwhelmed. It requires tools or techniques like *RST* and *RMM,* used daily, with consistent discipline, to increase Earth's *Chi* field passing through the body to sustain and improve health and *well-being.*

Two to five minute sessions of *RMM,* done at home or anywhere, throughout the day, represents an easy starting point. When the opportunity arises to commit to a half hour session or more daily the benefits are magnified. *RST* requires the interface of a certified therapist. Depending on one's health, or severity of disease, this may be as infrequently as monthly for tune-ups to daily, bi-weekly, or weekly. With clinical improvement the frequency of treatments can be reduced.

Wilhelm Reich-*Orgone* Energy

Dr. Wilhelm Reich was a psychoanalyst in the 1930's. He postulated the presence of a universal life force he called *Orgone* energy. He created what he called an *Orgone* box. This box was made of wood, lined with alternating layers of metal and wool. He also made a blanket with the alternating pattern of wool and metal.

Dr. Reich claimed that *Orgone* energy was para-magnetic and stimulated a healing, repair response in organic tissue. Placing part or all of the body wrapped in an *Orgone* blanket or box, would facilitate improved health outcomes.

I suspect that what Dr. Reich called *Orgone* energy represents a part of Earth's *Chi* energy. The metal demonstrates part of the *Orgone* field as electric or electro-magnetic. Was the *Orgone* field similar to the field identified in *Earthing?* Using wood and wool demonstrates part of the *Orgone* field as something other than electric. Was the *Orgone* field similar to the field identified in *grounding?*

Dr. Reich claimed that his *Orgone* energy was spontaneously generated within the box or around the blanket regardless of location. Would the *Orgone* field be enhanced if the blanket or box were utilized on a *grounded* surface?

Chi is more than an electro-magnetic energy *form*. The quality and characteristics of *Chi,* as spirit, extend and expand through many layers and levels both definable and indefinable. I believe Dr. Reich was tapping an energy more inclusive than that represented by electromagnetism. I view his work as developmental in relation to *RST.*

Our Five Primary Senses as a Trap

Compare our five primary senses with other animals on the planet. In terms of acuity, human senses are relatively dull. Compare human sight with eagles or owls. Compare human hearing with dogs. Compare human smell with elephants. What about human taste? It is definitely much better than other senses, on a relative scale. The sense of taste is unique, requiring taste buds, directly on the tongue, and the sense of smell combined. The human tongue has a much denser concentration of taste buds compared to most other animals. What about human touch? It is extremely refined when it comes to playing an instrument, painting, writing, typing or reading Braille.

The human sense of touch may be the most refined in the entire animal kingdom, or at least certainly one of the best. Touch is the primary sense used to define ourselves as a body and distinguish the border of self and non-self. Touch is also the primary sense that induces excess fascial twisting that may lock our consciousness into the body shell. It is also the primary sense to reverse this *process* and free us.

Our five primary senses are a major contributing and maintaining force, holding us from the perception of our true selves. As we come to understand this more fully, we are able to use the senses as they were intended, as a springboard to help release us, rather than bind us.

After we firmly establish that we are a body, we discover we are a gender; male or female. We discover we are a race; white, black, red or yellow. We discover language, a profound and wondrous tool that like our senses helps bind us and potentially free us at the same time. We discover and identify ourselves as a family, society, country, culture and create religious or political affiliations. All of these pieces together are *be-mi;* the body, ego, mind and identity. Eckhart Tolle popularized this phrase expressed as mind, body, ego, identity.

Just as the body is a shell, the ego, mind and identity are also shells or aspects of who we are rather than what we are. Who we are and who we become, is directly related to our life experiences and exposures relative to the factors of body, gender, race, language, family, society, culture, religion and politics. We are prone to think or perceive that who we are is ostensibly what we are; the who, is usually dis-connected and its expression as *be-mi* holds us back from the realization of our true self-essence. Who we are can be personally framed and understood in a functional *context* to support our connecting, waking up journey, as to what we are, as spiritual, *transcendent beings*. Part of the essential purpose of this book is to offer a template that can be used to make this shift.

The Heart Entrains the Brain

Voice, as language, is predominantly a medium through which we communicate from the *mind-brain*. This type of communication is generally derived from our awareness of self, as who we think we are. It is a reflection and projection of *be-mi*. The ability to use language, to project into another person's mind the image of an object is astounding. When I say tree, you see a tree in your mind's eye. The *form* of the tree may be different for different people but the image shared is universal and recognizable. In our capacity as a transmitter, language from the *mind-brain* is a projection of *out-flow*.

In our capacity as a receiver, voice, either as pure tones or language, may also be a medium for communication from the heart. Language from the heart is a reception of *in-flow*.

Research from the Institute of HeartMath (18) has demonstrated that the heart entrains the brain, exerting a controlling influence on it. This revolutionary concept reframes the brain's regulatory role in the body. The regulatory function that the heart exerts on the brain is related to the rhythmic nature of its beating.

Historically, the brain has been considered the master control organ, exerting critical regulatory functions for all other organs and systems of the body. Both the heart and brain exhibit a wave-pulse function.

Electrical readouts, in the form of an EEG for the brain and an EKG for the heart, demonstrate this wave-pulse phenomenon. The electrical magnitude of the heart's EKG is, by many factors, greater than the electrical magnitude of the brains EEG.

In a developing fetus the heart induces a rhythmic pulse, beat and wave at the earliest stages of fascial compartmental differentiation of organ specificity. The heart's pulse, beat, wave is the first primordial audible sound of the body. All further fascial compartmental organ differentiation and function is dependent on the primordial heart generated sound. It is sound functioning as the *cause* substrate that induces fascial membranes to coalesce into *forms.* These *forms* are the templates used to make all organs and parts of the body. The brain and nervous system are one of the last body systems to fully develop.

The premise of the heart's entrainment of the brain is defined as a dominant over-ride control mechanism that the heart exerts on the brain. Normal or optimal brain or central nervous system function is dependent on the pulse, beat, wave coming from the heart.

HeartMath research has demonstrated the ability of a changing EKG to influence and facilitate change in an EEG. The sound of the heart is a physical dimension manifestation of the primordial cosmic music of the spheres.

The sound, word, *shab* is the *cause* substrate crossing through the membrane between the *un-manifest nothing* dimensions into the worlds of manifestation.

Toning

Toning can use any vocal sound. The range, pitch and volume are variable. However, generally *toning* uses simple vowel sounds: A, E, I, O and U or any *mantra* such as: *Aum*, Baju, Hum or *Hu*. *Toning* can also be singing, using pure sounds or uplifting lyrics:

Row, row, row your boat,

Gently down the stream,

Merrily, merrily, merrily, merrily,

Life is but a dream.

What a delightful metaphor for life! Life in balance is in the flow, in the rhythm and the sound. To *be* in surrender to *Chi* as spirit. This is the stream manifest as living joyously. *Lila*; is the play of soul, it is *unconditional*, open and receptive, aware that life as we experience it in the physical dimension is a transitional reality.

This allows us to frame our experience in gratitude and humility, reflected from a simple children's nursery rhyme.

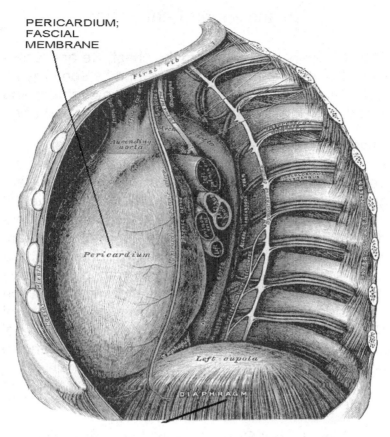

PERICARDIUM;
FASCIAL
MEMBRANE

Fig. 31

FASCIAL MEMBRANE; DIAPHRAGM &
PERICARDIUM

(Pericardium; fascial membrane around the heart
Diaphragm; thickened *fascia* separating organs of the
upper and lower abdominal cavity)

Rhythm-Heart-Beat-Sound

At birth, when we are held to the chest, we are reconnected to the beating of the heart and its soothing effect. This principle of rhythm, both as movement and sound, is crucial for equilibrium of mind, body and spirit.

Underlying the words that make up language is sound, specifically vocal sound. This sound, in and of itself, is a *transcendent* language, part of which is found in all languages universally. I use the acronym *USL;* universal sound language to identify or reference this *transcendent* vocal language. A cry, sigh, laugh, grunt, moan, wail, as well as baby goo, goos, gaa, gaas and daa daas, are all part of this *transcendent* language. I have defined *transcendent* as a linkage of divine connection and guidance. This is a link through all dimensions of *STEM; space-time,* energy and matter, across the final membrane that is the border, boundary between the *no-thing, un-manifest,* divine God realm and all worlds or dimensions of duality that are polarized and made manifest.

Pure Vocal Sound as a *Transcendent* Language; 6th Sense

The purest *form* of this *transcendent* language is vocal sound, as in the singing of pure tones or the use of *mantra. Mantra* is the use of specific vocal sounds to induce a *resonant harmonic* within the shell of the body. This changes the frequency and vibration in the physical body, influencing its *form* and function. It also affects the emotional, causal, mental, subconscious and spiritual bodies.

Use of this *transcendent* vocal language is the literal key to expand consciousness, experience divine presence and consciously cross through all dimensional layers of reality. With a commitment to mastery of *USL,* we can wake up. As we wake up, experiences follow and we remember our birthright, as *soul,* to travel freely across the last membrane, separating *no-thing* from everything. This allows us to *be* pure *cause,* no longer subject to the endless cycles of *cause* and effect. We can understand and choose our role of service with the divine; service to all life, all beings, all existence.

The human voice is a medium of communication. This is utilization of voice as a transmitter. When awakened it is a sixth sense. By definition, a sense is a means whereby we receive input or data. Our five primary physical senses are derived from actual body organs. The input or data coming to us from these physical sense organs bombard us continuously. They are subject to *mind-brain* interpretation but otherwise seem to be out of our conscious control.

The voice activated *as USL* is a medium for receiving input and data. Unlike our five primary senses that bind us to our physical *form* in *space-time* by receiving and perceiving data from the physical dimension only, our voice is capable of receiving and perceiving data from a frequency band wider than the physical. *USL* turns a key to catalyze this *transcendent* linkage. Sensory input that expands normal senses is a sixth sense. To see a ghost or apparition is an expanded sixth sense of vision. To feel a non-physical energy-force is an expansion of touch.

Hearing music, when there is none, is an expansion of hearing. Can we learn to activate or potentiate these abilities? *USL* functions as just such a tool.

The voice is unique, there is a clear pathway, a *free will* choice to engage it in its *transcendent form* as *USL*. This *form* opens the door into a divine linkage that further opens the door into an unlimited range of *transcendent* perception.

Resonant Sound Therapy

Resonant Sound Therapy or *RST* is a therapeutic modality I have developed. The full title of this modality is *resonant harmonic sound, modulated frequency and amplitude, fascial release therapy*. This therapy has evolved as a synthesis over twenty-five years of clinical practice as a Naturopathic physician and over thirty-five years of personal internal cultivation of *Chi* and meditation practices using *mantra* or vocal chanting.

RST has several levels of application. They range from clinical applications, utilized by a therapist with a patient to a variety of self-help modalities. These applications relate to balancing all aspects of life from the physical, emotional, mental and spiritual realms.

A primary application, in its clinical *form*, is made by having a patient make a vocal tone over which the practitioner makes a resonant vocal overtone. These tones can be very simple, to very complex. While humming a sound the chest vibrates. Other parts of the body vibrate as well.

When a practitioner hums with a patient, if that humming is *resonant*, it induces a body *harmonic*. The body is now vibrating in multiple frequencies simultaneously. This *harmonic* can occur with a single voice, but is easier to induce with more than one voice. If the vibration of the vocal cords is the fundamental tone, then the *harmonic* occurs as the vocal cords simultaneously vibrate in segments of halves, thirds, fourths and more.

Mathematically, each segment is an integral multiple of the frequency of the whole vocal cord. Each segment vibrates respectively twice, three times, four times, or in increasing multiples as fast as the whole vocal cord.

These variable and simultaneous sound frequencies are synchronized with physical contact and movement, initiated by the therapist to the patient that is both vibrational and rotational.

This vibrating, rotational movement, combined with the vocal sound, is what modulates or changes the frequency and amplitude of the fascial *Chi* interface. At this interface *RST* activates and potentiates release of fascial torque or twisting.

Fascial torque or twisting causes a disruption in the flow of *Chi* or energy through the body leading to imbalances. Understanding the function and role of *fascia* and how to release it is a key to *well-being*, healing and expanded consciousness.

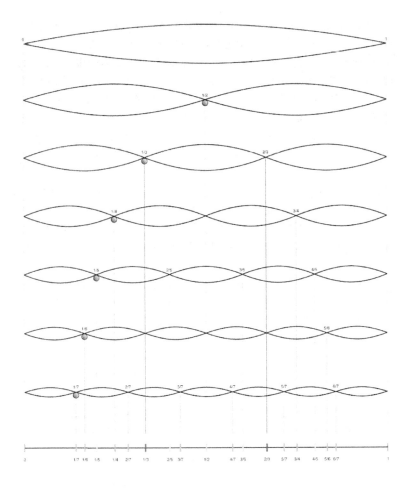

Fig. 32

SCALE OF HARMONICS

The top row shows the fundamental tone. Each next lower row shows how the tone is divided into additional partial segments: 1/2 tones, then 1/3, 1/4, 1/5, 1/6 and 1/7 tones. The visual quality of a dual spiral winding tighter and tighter is the fundamental *form* of *Chi* or life force energy flowing through the body.

Tuning Forks-Principle of *Resonance*

Sound is heard when a tuning fork is struck. The sound coming from this first tuning fork projects a vibratory wave in all directions. As this wave hits a second tuning fork, of the same note, resonance causes a sympathetic vibration that now induces the second tuning fork to vibrate and also make an audible sound. This is the principle of *resonance* in action. As both tuning forks resonate, their combined sound timbre or character makes overtones that create additional *harmonics*.

Voice is organic and capable of unique complex tonal variations, not reproducible by any machine. I use the term, organic, to define anything naturally occurring or derived from nature in its whole *form*. When something natural is adulterated, modified artificially, has a constituent extracted or is made completely synthetically, it is not organic. Although an extracted constituent, like a specific plant alkaloid may fundamentally be completely natural, its removal from the whole plant modifies the function or activity of both the plant and the isolated constituent. Using the current formal definition of organic, a natural constituent will be identified and acknowledged as organic. Based on my definition of organic, it will not.

An example to put this in perspective is looking at green tea. Green tea is an herb with a large body of scientific research identifying its constituents and properties. One constituent in green tea is caffeine. Research has shown that all the beneficial health promoting attributes of green tea are reduced when it is de-caffeinated.

It is as if the caffeine acts as a unifying and stabilizing bridge for the other components in the green tea. *The whole being greater than the sum of its parts* is a guiding principle integral to my definition of organic.

In the discipline of alternative medicine, one aspect is the branch of energy medicine. The essential essence inherent in all *forms* of energy medicine is frequency or vibration. This concept is predicated on the premise that everything is or has a unique frequency. When this frequency is in normal balance it promotes health and *well-being*. When the frequency is disrupted, there is an energy dis-equilibrium leading to symptoms and diseases. Most modern energy medicine is based on the development and utilization of machines that generate frequencies. There are many of these types of machines and more and more being developed. Currently, there is no clear consensus in the field of energy medicine, as to what the correct health promoting, disease preventing or reversing frequencies are. There may be specific frequencies that have universal applications, although the concept of some idealized list of such beneficial frequencies is questionable.

Just as no fingerprints are identical, no one has the exact same frequency print. This mandates greater individuation of therapy to optimize outcomes. Many frequency machines are capable of creating and developing this type of customized, personalized, energy treatment protocols. The price point of this machine technology is extremely variable, from less than one-hundred dollars to tens of thousands of dollars. The market of this machine technology is competitive, with claims and counter-claims of what really works.

Much of this technology may be effective but there is not enough objective research to adequately guide patients or therapists yet. Over time, this technology will improve and standards of effectiveness be implemented.

RST is a hands on, vocal, organic *process*. It is teachable and reproducible. Is it possible that this type of low-tech therapy can be as effective as the most sophisticated machines that will ever be produced? Is it possible that this type of organic human to human healing *process,* in time, will come to overshadow and outperform all machines?

In my clinical experience of treating many intractable conditions and terminal patients, *RST* has proven to be a uniquely effective and potent therapeutic tool. Our own internal, rather than external resources are an essential part of sustainable healing and expanding enlightenment. Many sound therapists utilize tuning forks, bowls, bells or a variety of sound induction machines in their clinical work. These are external tools and have definite therapeutic usefulness. None of these tools are necessary with *RST* but may be integrated on an individual practitioner basis. The beauty, clarity and simple yet complex tones of the human voice are not dependent on any external augmentation.

Humans have entered the technology and innovation era at an accelerated rate. The potential seems limitless. Due to this potential, our enthusiasm, and the novelty of this expansive technology, we have willingly entered into the first phase of a complex experiment.

It is interesting that there are so many books, movies and TV shows offering story lines that would have us pause, slow down, or just plain stop having an interface with technology. Where is this coming from? Is it fear, intuition, premonition, some combination of these, or something else?

Battlestar Galactica, Terminator and *Transformers* all warn us of dire consequences as machines develop *AI; artificial intelligence.* As *AI* is achieved, in all of these examples, the machines immediately know that humans are an inferior life *form* to be exterminated. Humans aren't even worthy of being kept as pets.

Currently, it seems, that popular belief and scientific evidence is that machine *AI* is both inevitable and imminent.

The TV series, *Revolution* is set in present time. The planetary power grid has failed or been turned off. Many contend that this type of catastrophic failure is possible. How dependent is the average human on current technology? If the plug was pulled, who would have the skill set to survive? The caveat, be careful of unbalanced reliance on technology. Basic planetary stewardship and skills of gardening and animal husbandry should be reintegrated into our basic educational systems.

It is viable and practical to find a balance between the natural world and technology. They need not be mutually exclusive. As the steep curve of technologic expansion progresses, finding and implementing this balanced interface is critical.

The warning from science, science fiction and fantasy is that if the necessary equilibrium is not established and maintained, our technology could be our undoing.

Using objects, tools or technology external to ourselves, can potentially augment rather than detract or distract us from our journey of awakening. The only way we can functionally use or ultimately benefit from any external object, tool or technology is to frame it *contextually,* relative to our awakening journey.

The usage of the word *contextually*, is defined as the most connected, functionally useful, uplifting and divinely guided space. The context: *to be in the world but not of it. We are not the body, the body is only a shell, we are soul.* This is literal, not figurative.

Our true home, or existence, is through the last membrane or edge separating, *STEM; space-time,* energy and matter from the *un-manifest no-thing* realm, home of *soul.* To cross this barrier requires that we actualize the awareness that all objects, tools and technology are here as mediums of learning. The primary lesson, is for us to choose non-attachment. It is our attachment to objects, tools or technology that binds us to them and consequently to the polarized dimensions of *STEM.* The *context* is to identify, understand, interface and utilize mastery of *form* and function through surrender, release and detachment.

Fascial Membrane-Source of Increased Body Awareness

During physical contact with a patient, the vocal harmonic induced from both their voices is transmitted through the body. The contact creates a dampening effect. This physical interface between the patient and therapist is the foci where the *harmonic* wave is concentrated.

The dampening effect increases subjective awareness to specific areas of the body. This increased specific body awareness is transmitted between the patient and therapist. The medium for this increased subjective awareness is the fascial membrane. This increase in body perceptual awareness is central to the patient's ability to release and unwind their own *fascia,* as well as the therapist's ability to function as a guide to help the patient achieve fascial release. Initially it is common to have a low level of conscious subjective fascial body awareness. With self-practice, using *RMM* and ongoing *RST* sessions, this sensitivity increases. Even if a patient's fascial release is unconscious, during early treatments, the therapist is able to feel and confirm the release. Increased body awareness is partially due to the sense of the relative position of different body parts to each other, known as proprioception. Sound and touch combined improves the ability to find and release the fascial membrane.

A patient with osteomyelitis of the right foot, had undergone multiple surgeries and bone grafts. After one treatment with *RST* he was able to feel his foot for the first time in many years.

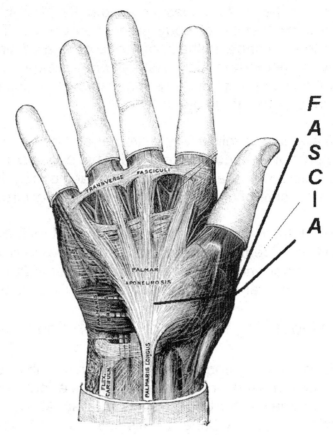

Fig. 33

FASCIA OF HAND

This image shows the first superficial layer of *fascia* under the skin. This layer surrounds and encapsulates all the muscles. This is the first layer that we are able to feel and differentiate from the outside or surface of the body.

Through the *RST process*, as we identify this first layer, a new awakening of body perception occurs. This is due to the connectedness of *fascia* as one continuous woven membrane. The natural progression of *RST* awakens a perception, as a simultaneous feeling of the entire surface of the body.

We are able to follow *fascia* deeper and deeper as every part of the body is identified. This capacity to find, feel and unwind *fascia*, from the surface of our skin, to the very core of our bone marrow, is a natural birthright.

This ability induces not only a perceptual shift that allows us to remember our birth, but is a gateway to a much older and deeper remembering that is *transcendent* of the transitory states of physical life and death.

Modulating Frequency as Vibrating Spiral

The modulating frequency is based on the observation that *Chi*, a synonym for Ki or Qi; the life force energy that animates the body, travels in a spiral, with a vibrating frequency pattern. This spiral has a parallel in *Kundalini yoga*. (19) During an *RST* treatment the amplitude of the spiral is varied, as a patient's limb or a more localized part of the body is moved. Amplitude can be visually represented as the peaks and valleys of a wave. It is a measurement of height or distance. The frequency, or speed, is adjusted by physically transmitting a shaking or trembling vibration from therapist to patient.

This allows the therapist to find *Chi* as it flows, both tactilely and visually. Twisting of *fascia* induces blockage. By varying the *resonant harmonic*, as well as amplitude and frequency of both voice and physical contact, *fascia* unwinds, restoring *Chi* to unrestricted flow and full function.

This *process* induces a state of symbiosis. The boundary of the patient's fascial membrane becomes more permeable, generating a link between their *fascia* and the therapist. Once the link is established, the therapist can modify the spiral amplitude and vibrating frequency, combined with the *resonant harmonic* sound, to act as a guide, to help the patient accelerate release and unwinding of their fascial membrane. *Chi,* transmitted through the Earth from one body to another, potentiates the re-establishing of an equilibrium state. The potential is to allow *Chi* to flow without restriction, through all layers of *fascia*, to open the door from within for the patient's personal healing and expanded consciousness.

Subjective Experience

Chi charge is on and embedded in fascial membrane. In this journey, I have made many discoveries through personal observation and experience. These observations are paradoxical and at times have been personally confusing or disorienting. As observable patterns evolved, I entered a place where I recognized that any limited perception or thought was self-induced. The premise that we are all bound by the limits of our five primary senses is only true because we accept it as truth. This starts to put things in a whole new light.

What is or is not true or real? Einstein proved that we live in a *relative universe*. (20) Let me reframe this with an esoteric definition*: as we see it, say it, feel it, think it, know it, so it is.* Are there things completely outside of our personal relative perception that are just true? I hope by the end of this book that you will have a clearer perception and a more expanded view to answer this question for yourself.

It is a novel premise that we can gather information, knowledge and expanded awareness through an internal rather than external medium. Western culture tries to make it clear that legitimate facts, truths and figures are outside ourselves. Science is the new religion and all answers will come from this external all powerful source. Science has helped us expand our perception, knowledge and awareness. It is an external tool, one for us to use, understand and frame *contextually*. This book is not about limitations or restrictions. It is not about making any tool or awareness right or wrong. This book is an offering from me to you to share a journey, a journey to help you refine and expand your own personal perceptions and world view.

The discovery of the initial qualities and location of *Chi* is the foundational framework that led to observations about the nature, function and purpose of both *fascia* and *Chi*.

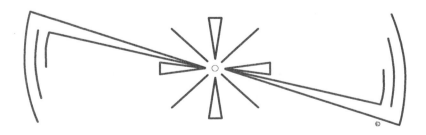

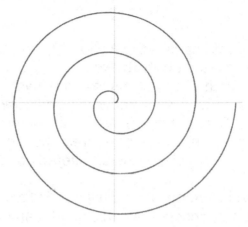

Fig.34

ARCHIMEDEAN SPIRAL

The above spiral, mathematically described by Archimedes, (21) a famous Greek mathematician, physicist,
engineer, inventor and astronomer is a simple graphic
representation demonstrating how *Chi* flows through
the body. As a two dimensional construct it does not
reflect the more detailed model necessary for a deeper
understanding and awareness of *Chi* flow. Another perceptual level demonstrates *Chi* flow as a conical helix.
The differential from a simple spiral to a conical helix
demonstrates initial perceptual levels of *Chi* moving
through a body.

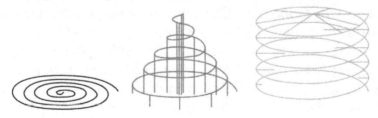

Fig. 35

SPIRAL- CONICAL HELIX- HELIX

117

Whirling Dervish

Ancient systems like *Chi Kung* (22) or *Tai Chi Chuan* (23) cultivate the ability to experience *Chi*-energy passing through the body. In *Sufism*, the mystical branch of Islam, there is a sect known as the *whirling dervish* (24) sect. They practice a system of spiraling, rotational movement combined with sacred chanting capable of inducing a state of expanded, altered consciousness.

In codified systems like *Tai Chi* or *Sufism*, the guiding masters or teachers may imply that many years of diligent work are necessary before any significant spiritual or healing progress can be attained. *RST* and *RMM* decode, demystify and accelerate personal experience of *Chi*. We remember that healing and enlightenment come from *being unconditional in the moment.*

Bio-Energetic Synchronization Technique

Dr. Milton Morter developed an elegant and simple system he called B.E.S.T. ; *Bio-Energetic Synchronization Technique.* (25) Other systems of fascial work include basic massage, Osteopathic, *Strain-Counter-strain* and *Cranial Sacral*, (26) *Trager,* (27) *Feldenkrais*, (28) Yoga, *Chi Gong*, *Tai Chi*, acupressure and acupuncture, Chiropractic techniques like *AK; applied kinesiology* and *Network* Chiropractic, *Polarity*, (29) *Rolfing,* (30) *Jin Shin Jyutsu*, (31) *Reiki*, (32) *EFT; emotional freedom technique*, (33), Rudolf Steiner's *Eurythmy* and Elizabeth Keyes *toning.* All are effective in their own right. This list is not intended to be comprehensive or exclusionary.

RST, is a product of my own inner *process*. It is not derived from any of the systems or *forms* listed above, yet shares common elements. In these various systems the following elements may or may not be included; external touch, passive motion, self-movement, rhythmic motion and sound whether vocal or not. *RST* integrates vocal *resonance* and *harmonics* with rhythm, touch and motion as an integrated whole.

Chi Blockage as Fascial Torque
Definition: Charge as Energetic Projection

Chi blockage is caused by a twisting or torque of the fascial membrane due to a physical, emotional, mental, subconscious or spiritual injury or trauma. Fascial torque induced from injury or trauma at any of these levels in a balanced, optimally functioning human is self-limiting and spontaneously reverses. This reversal or unwinding of *fascia* re-establishes energetic equilibrium. With injuries or traumas that manifest with permanent body, organ or system damage, the natural energetic outcome will still spontaneously revert to an equilibrium state. This equilibrium state does not automatically correct or cure anything. It does activate the natural *process* of *healing.*

Comparing the terms cure and *heal* clarifies energetic equilibrium. Cure is a *process* that engages a battle with the intent to fight and win against the evil that is a disease or any negatively perceived injury, trauma or imbalance. In this model, disease as the enemy must be destroyed.

This places us in an adversarial role in which the outcome we are striving for is framed as trying to get what we *think* we want. Consider this: *in a war, there are no winners, ever.*

Healing, or *Nature Cure*, refers to a *process* whereby we actually get what we *need*, not just what we think we want. In this model, neither cancer nor any disease is evil nor the enemy.

The dis-ease *process* offers us a window, as an opportunity, to learn, grow and develop more compassion and tolerance for ourselves and others. In this *process* the dis-ease or symptoms may or may not go away. There is a fundamental shift in our awareness and understanding. *When in dynamic balance, what we want and what we need become synonymous.* In the example of a situation where a disease or injury manifests permanent body damage, with *healing* the damage may remain.

With *healing* comes awareness and the ability to authentically be grateful for the gift of experience that the divine has given. We suspend any projections of judgment, whether toward self, inward or toward others, outward, as shame, blame or victimhood. We release any negatively charged emotions linked to any perceived negative event. Charge here is defined as an energetic projection that is oriented in a relative *context* identifying good versus bad. This charge always has an emotional hook due to personal framing of experience in this relative context.

For the emotion to be a hook, we couple an image in our mind's eye, either a memory or projection of the future with sadness, fear, pain, anger, lust, greed, vanity, or any other *form* of attachment. Any image that is coupled with any of the above negative emotions, induces the charge that makes an interference pattern, twisting *fascia* and disrupting *Chi* flow.

Definition: Charge as Poles in Energy System

Chi is an energy *form* of balanced positive and negative charges. Charge here is identified as the two poles in a polarized energy system. Electricity has a positive and negative pole. The charge associated with *Chi*, like electricity, has no correlation with good or bad.

Yin-Yang

We live in a polarized universe of positive and negative charge, expressed as the positive, Yang, masculine, active, upward, hot, white, bright, light, motion, expanding pole and the negative, Yin, feminine, passive, downward, cold, black, dark, still, contracting pole. To quote Annemarie Colbin, from one of my favorite cookbooks, *The Book of Whole Meals, The Yin-Yang principle is a value-free system of classifying universal phenomena into pairs of opposites…They both spring from the Undifferentiated One, or Infinity; together interplaying in various directions, amplitudes and speeds, they cause all visible and invisible phenomena…they do not remain still but continuously change from one into the other, attracting each other when they're most different, repelling each other when they are more alike* (34).

Chi is recognized as the manifestation or result of the properties of Yin and Yang interacting on each other.

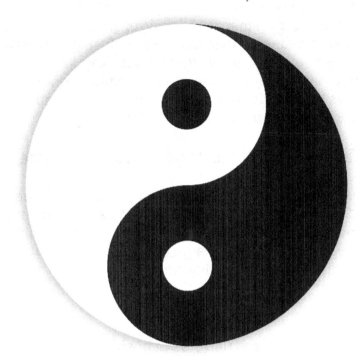

Fig. 36

YIN-YANG SYMBOL

Everything exists as a balanced interchange between opposites. Everything is either expanding or contracting at any particular time. A seed germinates and grows in its expanding phase. As maximum expansion is achieved, the balanced tipping point is reached and the contraction cycle starts. The plant withers and eventually dies. This is true of plants, animals, humans, planets, suns and the universe. To equate expansion as good and contraction as bad is naive, predicated on an incomplete knowledge or awareness of their balanced and essential interchanges.

Annemarie Colbin further offers, *too much expansion and we fly off into space, too much contraction and we become dried up dwarfs. (35)* Without understanding, taking the properties of Yin and Yang at their extremes, they may seem either good or bad. Good and bad are human mental constructs, coming from a limited or biased perspective and perception. The common cultural, social, religious foundation, framing good and bad as divine or God derived uncontestable absolutes, if examined from a neutral objective perspective, are readily identified as being derived from *be-mi;* body, ego, mind and identity. This explains how and why different religions disagree or are in conflict relative to their interpretation or belief in what is good or bad.

Common to all religions, philosophies and moral, ethical codes, a *golden thread* of commonality joins all of them. Is it probable or possible that this *golden thread* may be the closest, mentally derived approximation, to divine or Godly truth or will?

Is there another level of information or guidance that *transcends* belief or mental abstractions? Is such a level accessible only on an individual basis, through diligence and effort, into a *transcendent* linkage of *self-discovery, awakening and healing?* The answers lie within. When our personal discovery and awareness, is in alignment with others, we can rejoice and celebrate together. When such discovery or awareness is not in alignment with others, we can still choose to rejoice and celebrate our diversity and individuality together.

God's preeminent quality is *unconditional* love. We are all the children of the divine. We are all accepted without reservation. There is no divine hesitation. There is no judgment. There is no list of good or bad that defines whether God accepts us or not.

Macrobiotics

Macrobiotics (36) is a dietary system utilizing the principles of Yin and Yang, in which all of the properties previously ascribed to Yin and Yang remain constant, except contraction and expansion which are reversed. In Macrobiotics, sugar, represents the extreme of Yin as expansion, salt, represents the extreme of Yang as contraction. Macrobiotic practitioners and followers use the concepts of expansion or contraction to identify food properties and generally avoid the terms Yin and Yang.

This is a prime example of our relative universe in action; depending on our language, social and cultural upbringing, as well as education, we have profoundly different world views. Which is right and which is wrong? It is human nature to presume that what we have been taught or believe is a definitive framework from which we can judge or place value on persons, places, things and thoughts. Become self-aware, refrain from dogmatic or strong views or opinions about anything. Applying the principles of Yin and Yang to these views offers us the ability to take the charge, emotional hook, judgment or presumed value out of the equation.

Interference Patterns

When energy disruption of *Chi* occurs due to a charge that torques *fascia*, it becomes a foci; focal point, that secondarily induces a symptom complex which may have physical, emotional, mental, subconscious or spiritual manifestations. If not brought into energetic equilibrium, these symptoms may progress into formal pathology or disease. A charge in *space-time* that is conditional, is framed in a relative context identifying good versus bad, which induces an energetic interference pattern that torques the body's fascial membrane. This disrupts the normal balanced positive and negative energy flow of *Chi* or life force.

The More We Know, The More We Know, The Less We Know

Cycles go from the simple, to the more complex, to the more complex and back full circle to the simple. Increasing levels of complexity elucidated in any system, increase awareness and understanding up to a point, then the system collapses and implodes and the cycle is renewed. *The more we know, the more we know, the less we know.* Questions breed more questions. Prevailing scientific enquiry, predominantly using deconstruction as dissection, increases information relating to complexity and detail. General belief is the more details we discover relative to anything, the more it will be understood. The paradox from the axiom above stipulates the opposite.

First there is a mountain, then there is no mountain, then there is. This spiritual principle popularized by the folk singer Donovan in his song, *There is a Mountain,* (37) reflects the stages of spiritual awakening in which things are first seen as superficial objects; what is defined as superficial is also called the mundane. This level has the highest density or concentration of physical matter; first there is a mountain. Then the mountain is seen in a fuller, deeper *context*. The *context,* as a spiritual awakening, is a direct experiential link of perception. This link leads from the tactile, visible state of matter, through the microscopic, molecular, atomic and sub-atomic levels into pure energy; then there is no mountain. In the integration stage, awareness and perception of the mountain melds the mundane with the *transcendent;* then there is, (*a mountain again.*)

This example, exemplifying the nature of paradox, demonstrates the *process* of perceptual change from the contracted to the expanded, to the contracted, to the more expanded. There is a place of knowing, being, experiencing that eludes layers of complexity, that is inherently simple, that is accessible from a space that is neither linear nor mind driven.

Parable of Blind Men and Elephant-Paradox

In the parable of *The Blind Men and the Elephant*, (38) three blind men approach an elephant. One of them bumping into the leg cries out, *surely the elephant is like a mighty tree*. Another, grabbing the trunk states that the former is mistaken, *for truly the elephant is like a snake.*

126

The third, grabbing the elephant's tail says to the other two, *how can you be so misled, an elephant is clearly like a rope?* The delightful part of this parable is that the reader, having the proverbial bird's eye view can recognize the great paradox; all of them are right and yet all of them are wrong.

Perceptual Levels of Matter

Matter perceived through our five senses is tangible. A pencil held in our hand is smooth and solid. If a tool is used to augment perception, like a magnifying glass, the seemingly smooth surface appears rough and pitted. Understanding what and how a magnifying glass works, allows for simultaneously acknowledging that both perceptions of reality are correct, with no conflict. Under a microscope, the increased magnification of the pencil shows even more imperfections. Without the aid of a magnifying glass or microscope, could you be convinced of the simple truths they reveal about the surface of the pencil?

Molecular Level

What is true or real? There is an inherent danger in accepting external authority. It makes us less independent, self-sufficient and more complacent. In chemistry things are made up of units or pockets of matter called molecules. As a function of *common knowledge,* (39) this is readily accepted as true, despite little or no personal subjective confirmation or understanding.

No molecules of an original material can be found in a chemical analysis of any solution diluted beyond *Avogadro's number,* ~ 6.0 x 10 to the 23rd power. The information derived from the molecular level is presumed as true and correct but only represents a specific, narrow bandwidth of data. This expanded level of information does not negate the physical or microscopic perceptual level, it is additive. It adds from the contracted, physical, to the expanded, molecular, to the more expanded, atomic.

Atomic Level

At the atomic level, energy and matter are synonymous. From Einstein's equation:

$$E=mc^2$$

Energy equals mass times the speed of light squared. The speed of light is 299.7 km/s (kilometers per second) or 186,000 miles/second. Most of us casually take these facts for granted, accepting an external authority for proof or verification. Acceptance of such an external authority is viewed as benign. This suggests that no harm or negative consequence can be associated with such a view. We're happy to be the recipients of electricity, airplanes and nuclear energy. If something goes wrong or breaks, someone else can fix it. The choice to utilize modern technology comes with a price.

Technology affords us more freedom and independence in one way, but in a profound and fundamentally different way, it makes us more dependent and less self-sufficient.

Matter is Mostly Empty Space

Matter from the atomic level is mostly empty space. How empty? According to modern physics, if we were to compress all physical matter on this planet to its extreme, the entire planet would be no larger than a baseball! If the *Big Bang Theory* is validated, than the entire physical universe came from one infinitesimally small speck. This parallels the premise of everything, coming from *no-thing*. The premise that all physical matter manifests through the membrane separating the *un-manifest* from the manifest. The conceptualization of Earth, as a ball of compressed matter, being the size of a baseball would be a gross over exaggeration, under these circumstances.

What is experienced through the five primary senses, is very different from the way things really are. This last statement is a value judgment. Isn't the way things really are, the way they are, as perceived through our five primary senses? Given the obvious limitations of physical sensory perception, the way things really are is much more than what is perceived through the senses exclusively.

Physical matter, from the *context* of matter, as perceived and experienced through our senses seems stable. Stability here is identified as un-moving and having a high level of physical density. Matter in the broader context, including the atomic perceptual level is also energy. This energy is neither un-moving nor physically dense. The energy qualities of matter, perceived from the *context* of our senses only, are limited and inaccurate.

Matter, from the *context* of energy, is neither un-moving nor does it have a high level of physical density. Matter perceived physically, or matter understood as energy, both represent aspects or qualities attributable to matter. The matter level is more limited and contracted. The energy level is less limited and more expanded. The expanded does not negate the contracted, it is merely additive.

The energy state of matter is often depicted as protons and electrons spiraling around the nucleus of an atom. This is actually a theoretical perspective, derived partly through reproducible experimentation and partly as a mathematical extrapolation. It is important to remember that this depiction of energy, is not some definitive absolute truth. It no longer represents the current scientific data base. Super Colliders are machines able to accelerate atomic particles approaching the speed of light and shatter them. This technology has demonstrated the inadequacy and overly simplistic perspective of atoms merely being a nucleus with spiraling electrons and protons.

The Secret

The book and movie, *The Secret*, (40) suggests that we can create, influence or modify our own lives, health and future by utilizing the power of projecting positive *thoughts, images* and *feelings.* This concept is ancient and has been taught, practiced and written about, in one *form* or another, since the dawn of mankind.

It has been said that history repeats itself. This repetition is not exacting in *form* but the general content is the same. These repetitive cycles occur in the broader, big picture, historical *context* as well as on an individual, personal, experiential basis. The repetitive cycles always reflect specific patterns of content. The presence of the repeating patterns is not abstract but actual. This is a mechanism that the universe or divine uses to offer us, as essence or *soul,* an opportunity to identify and implement a part of the *mechanics of causation.*

It is up to us as *soul* to recognize the repeating pattern. Any experience with a repeating motif is the universe or divine attempting to alert us of an area in our life where we are blocked, and where a lesson is to be learned. The block is a direct effect of reacting in a conditional way to the repeating motif. The reaction is either a linkage of negative emotional charge or mental projection judgment. The lesson is to recognize the pattern and then consciously choose to *be unconditional* and stop reacting.

Remaining hypervigilant, identifying and responding to specific repetitive patterns, *unconditionally,* the universe responds by accelerating the frequency of these repetitive cycles. This enhances our ability to more consistently act and function as *cause* rather than effect. This allows us to actualize control of our own destiny as cause, which is our birthright as *soul.* When the lesson is learned, the repetitive cycle is extinguished. This is a benchmark of *soul's* mastery of *causation mechanics.*

As effect, our destiny controls us. It is our tenacious, unwavering commitment and insistence of self as *be-mi*; body, ego, mind and identity, that perpetuates our state or condition as effect.

For a contextual example let's compare the definitions of curing versus *healing.* To induce a cure, activation of the principles of positive *thought, feeling* and *action* must be engaged, driven by self-will as personal intent. To induce *healing*, our *thought, feeling* and *action* must be in alignment with divine guidance. This is a function of *thy will* or God's will as divine acceptance.

Waking up, we come to a deeper understanding of the power that can be manipulated on our behalf. As a function of self-will, through practice, we can actualize the manifestation of whatever we want. The more powerful we become, the easier it is to control or manipulate anything. This is the discovery and use of the power of one's self or personal will that links us to manifesting desires. I define 'cure' in the context of a projected desire. This is part of the natural progression of *soul* waking up, and not yet *soul* fully awakened.

Projections, as desires, induce a cycle of energetic imbalance in which we become the effect of our own causation. As effect, we are bound in a repetitive cycle that is a virtual loop of specific repeating patterns. The result of our seemingly positive projections demonstrate their effectiveness. The short term gain generated from our desire is like an ice-berg. Projections of our desires that generate personal gain, are symbolized as the portion of the ice-berg that can be seen. Our perception is that it is safe, our belief is that we are deserving.

This gives us a false sense of entitlement and justifies our projected desires.

The hidden part of the ice-berg, that is dangerous and destructive, is the consequence or effect of our seemingly positive projections if linked with negative emotions and judgments.These projections are desires, whether for self or others, linked with emotions like sadness, fear or anger and judgments like shame or blame. These projections induce a block, as a consequence of the desire, whether it is fulfilled or not.

Our ability to cognitively understand, and then act differently, *unconditionally,* is dependent on our vigilance in identifying the repetitive cycles the universe places in our perceptual path. Paradoxically, the less aware we are of the *mechanics of causation*, the longer the linear interval between these repeating cycles. As the cycle interval becomes longer we lose the ability to recognize the *cause* and effect relationship and risk being caught in a potentially endless loop as effect. The slightest glimmer, awareness or insight of a specific repetitive pattern, offers an opportunity to grab on to the divine guiding link. The challenge is to hold on and not be thrown off or distracted. If the divine link is lost or broken, the cycle of effect can be relentless.

It is up to us to make and maintain our personal link with divine guidance. The power or ability to make this connection is within each and every one of us. It is our personal responsibility and discipline to engage the active tools available to us and make this a reality.

H*ealing* comes when there is no resistance. Total and absolute surrender, trust and acceptance are essential. All projected *thoughts, feelings* and *actions* are released into the river of spirit. There can be no attachment to outcomes. Attachment drives the power back to my will or self-will. We are bound yet again. Synchrony between my will; what I want and *thy will;* what I need, must be established and maintained. In this synchronous state, we are *cause*. Refining our understanding and utilization of this *process* is important. Discrimination is crucial. This is *soul* awakened, operating through *causation mechanics.*

Ground Hog Day

In the movie, *Ground Hog Day*, (41) Bill Murray plays a character caught in a loop repeating the same day over and over. As he comes to the realization that what seems to be occurring, is in fact occurring, he makes a valiant effort to control, or change it by doing things differently. He attempts to change things by changing or controlling external events. Despite his actions and confidence that what he is doing will work, he discovers that the daily recurrent theme remains intact. This causes him to engage in more and more desperate attempts to change things, hoping to extricate himself from this loop.

Surrender (Acceptance) Resistance

A definition of insanity is doing the same thing over and over, expecting a different result. In *Ground Hog Day*, Bill Murray eventually realizes that his efforts are in vain.

Further attempts at manipulation of external events are useless. This place of *surrender* is a critical step in the awakening *process*. *Surrender* allows us to open awareness and realize that things or events happening outside ourselves are not what actually affect or control us. We start to recognize and consider another possibility. This possibility has entered our consciousness, as a direct result of our vigilance in identifying a repetitive cycle with a specific patterned content. This is a recognition of a divine guidance interface.

The action step that demonstrates understanding and a functional application of *process* or life control, *causation mechanics*, is changing the internal view, perspective or reaction to any external object or situation. The causation power control is from the inside, out and not from the outside, in. Bill Murray's character decides to stop trying to change the external situation and instead begins to change his internal attitude, a change to acceptance rather than resistance.

With resistance, we are in the victim role, with acceptance, we enter the non-victim role. This inner change breaks the repetitive cycle loop of experience that Bill Murray's character has been caught in, and the movie ends. Bill's character is now able to enter into a new and different day. This is the beginning of control as *cause*, no longer effect.

As We See It, So It Is

Things, external to us, influence or affect us. Our inability to change or control these things reinforces this perception.

The one thing we can definitely control or change in every situation is our response or reaction. Imagine your house burning to the ground. Although we can speculate how we might react to such a situation, until we experience it that speculation is only conjecture. In our mind's eye we can identify a variety of optional reactions.

At the negative extreme, we see ourselves arriving home and being overwhelmed with shock and disbelief. We fall on our knees sobbing uncontrollably, thinking everything we value and cherish is gone. Life is unfair and capricious. We are victims in an unjust world. At this extreme, either we commit suicide or play this memory tape of pain and suffering so consistently that we end up in a mental institution unable to function for the remainder of our life.

At the other end of the spectrum, we arrive home, observe the condition of our property and acknowledge with gratitude that we are alive and well. Our lost belongings are only objects, which we know we cannot take across the great divide between life and death. We pick up a shovel, proceed to cleanup and rebuild. We choose to move on with our life.

A Gift from Spirit

As spirit would have it, my family and I were gifted with this very experience. Note my reference to this experience being a gift. I believe there are no accidents, no coincidences, and no mistakes. All experiences *are* *learning* experiences.

136

The choice we have every moment with every experience, is to *be* conditioned by it; reacting to it, or not *be* conditioned by it; not reacting to it. Everyone shares these two fundamental choices in relation to every life experience or event.

Many gifts came through my family's experience with this fire. My family was home when the fire started and no one was harmed. When this incident occurred we were having some serious behavioral problems with our two sons. Having to pull together as a family, to nurture and support each other, as well as having to live in close quarters, helped us all understand and appreciate each other. We shared the gratitude of our mutual safety and the value and importance of relationships rather than our belongings, which are transitory.

The Cup Half Empty or Half Full

We all share the ability to see the world with our cup half empty or half full. Given that we really do have *free will,* why would any of us ever choose to see the world or our lives as half empty?

As Eckhart Tolle describes in his book, *A New Earth Awakening to Your Life's Purpose*, (42) we come to believe and accept that we are our *mind, body, ego, identity*. These are the parameters we use to create our personal world view, to identify our value system and develop judgments relative to a codified framing of what we believe or think is right or wrong, good or bad. With this value, judgment system in place, we are now able to look at ourselves, both literally, as in a mirror, as well as figuratively.

In the mirror, we can compare our body to TV and magazine commercials of what true and accepted beauty is. By choosing to use this culturally created artificial reference point, and perceiving our own body and features as similar to this cultural ideal, it may flatter our ego. The opposite reaction of self-reflection may reinforce a negative judgment of ourselves as neither meeting, nor ever being able to approach this artificial ideal of beauty. Minimally, this has the potential to generate an inferiority complex.

Now we are able to expand our comparison of self in relation to a host of variables we frame as desirable or not. We become drawn into the necessity of using a system of value, judgment to compare ourselves to everybody and everything. We compare our possessions, homes, educations, schools, jobs, wives, children and friends.

Under these circumstances we are unlikely to ever be happy, content or satisfied. We can't and won't let go. Life is struggle and competition. It is because of this self framing, that we are able to choose or perceive our lives as half full or empty.

The symbolic cup, we perceive as half full or half empty, is the same cup with the same fluid level either way. It is not things, people, places, events or circumstances that limit or bind us in the loop of effect. Outer appearances and experiences suggest the opposite. Any of us can look at our life or others around us and confidently see how age, health, economic strata and numerous other variables are effecting, influencing, limiting and controlling us.

Our life is a reflection of the inherent paradox of the universe and existence.

The effect of these external things or circumstances does not determine or control our ability to choose gratitude, acceptance and be *unconditional.* In this space we neither judge self nor others. We choose to refrain from projecting either negative emotions or thoughts.

Being cause has nothing to do with the power to control or change external things or events, it has everything to do with letting go and letting God. To be *unconditional* is to be *detached. Detached* is not separated, cold and un-caring. *Detached* is free from attachments that bind and limit us. It is the most accepting, empathetic, warm, connected, caring and *unconditionally* loving space we can *be* in. As *cause*, the cup is neither half full nor empty, it is just a cup.

Things or circumstances may affect us but only our attachment to them binds us. It is critical to understand how attachment manifests. It is bi-directional. Strong desire for a thing, circumstance or outcome, binds us to the degree that we must have it. Strong desire to not have a thing, circumstance or outcome, binds us to the degree that we must avoid it.

We may or may not be able to control or change external events or circumstances. Either way, this level of seeming control or manipulation is not essence or *soul* functioning as *cause.* What we can control and change at all times, in all circumstances, is our *attitude, attention* and *awareness.*

Chi in All its *Forms* is Expressed through a Wide Bandwidth

Frequencies of light, sound, spirit, energy that make up *Chi* extend through a wide bandwidth. A bandwidth is the width of the range or band of an established block of frequencies.

As an example, on a specific transmission medium an electronic signal, like a radio bandwidth will be expressed in terms of the difference between its highest and lowest frequency signal components. A portion of the bandwidth of *Chi* can be perceived through the five primary senses. Humans have significant perceptual limitations relative to many qualities of this bandwidth, compared to other animal species. These limitations are understood and have been well documented.

Despite our intellectual acceptance of these facts, emotionally and perceptually, we often believe that what we perceive is all there is. This limited perception creates a built in bias that makes it difficult for us to accept the possibility and probability that reality may be larger or more expanded than the limited range of our physical senses.

It also makes it difficult for us to consider, let alone access, an expanded range of physical senses or other non-physical perceptual capabilities, that are actually available to humans as well.

Other parts of the bandwidth of *Chi,* we perceive with the augmentation of scientific equipment. The use of chemistry, *Newtonian* physics, microscopes, oscilloscopes and other tools demonstrate parts of a relative truth and prove that these even more expanded bandwidths exist. Most of us are not scientists and have little or no direct exposure to or use of scientific equipment. Despite this, we still fundamentally accept this expanded band-width of reality, based on what scientists tell us or demonstrate with their magical technology.

The prior problem bias of experiential and perceptual limitations is now magnified. Despite this, from an intellectual level, we suspend the evidence of our senses. This creates a dynamic tension. Subconsciously our tenuous grasp of reality is weakened. Often in the struggle to maintain any semblance of equilibrium we embrace a melding of science, religion and philosophy.

At its best, this gives us some modest sense of stability, purpose and meaning. It often allows us to function within the accepted familial and social norms or standards of our culture. On the surface, all seems well. Our essence, as *soul,* has an awareness that the mask of *be-mi;* body, ego, mind and identity is a thin veil, ready to be pierced at any moment. At its worst, the dynamic tension, conflict and confusion, is overwhelming. This may manifest as emotional and mental psychoses. This is the prime force that drives aberrant behaviors that manifest as harm to self or others.

In examining the band-width that encompasses all levels or aspects of *Chi,* two portions identified are those perceived through physical senses and those augmented with scientific equipment. Expanding beyond the realm of basic *Newtonian* physics and the limits of chemistry, microscopes and oscilloscopes, the domain of *Quantum* and *General Relativity* physics is entered. Some aspects of these *forms* of physics can be verified or quantified with physical experiments and machine technology. Some aspects remains theoretical. This level of science is even further removed from normal daily experiences.

It is essentially even more magical and less understandable, yet again, we blithely nod and bow our heads to the science gurus. More theoretical physics, like *String* and *Chaos theory*, have no current physical counterparts and are purely mathematical extrapolations. How does the average person relate to or understand any of these levels?

The prior problem, bias of experiential and perceptual limitations, is now magnified even more. Despite this, from an intellectual level, we continue to suspend the evidence of our senses. This creates even more dynamic tension. This tension manifests in the physical body as fascial twisting. It is critical for this tension to be released and a higher order of energetic equilibrium established. This equilibrium is established as layer after layer of *fascia* unwinds.

RST not only offers a mechanism for physical, emotional and mental health and *well-being*, it is also a tool to link our physical *fascia,* through *resonant harmonic* frequencies, with energetic membranes of less and less matter and more and more energy. This shifts and expands our bandwidth of perception well beyond the physical senses. This expanded perceptual bandwidth allows us to experientially reconcile physical sensory limitations with all *Newtonian, Quantum, General Relativity, String* and *Chaos* based physics both experimental and theoretical.

Other parts of the bandwidth of *Chi* we perceive as a function of a higher order of perception that is *transcendent.* This *transcendent* perception is independent of physical, emotional or mental mediators. It is spiritual. It is a divine linkage.

It comes from across the final membrane, from *nothing* to everything, from the inside, out, beyond *STEM;* *space-time*, energy and matter. This level is experiential and the birthright of *all* humans and is available to us through the use of *internal* tools such as *RST.*

TCM-Traditional Chinese Medicine and Acupuncture

In *TCM*-Traditional Chinese Medicine, (43) there are twelve primary and two extra acupuncture meridians through which *Chi* or energy passes. These channels are generally presumed to have no direct physical structure associated with them, however, their presence is verifiable with sensitive equipment picking up differing electrical potentials on the surface of the skin.

Chi flows from one meridian to the next, alternating between Yin and Yang meridians. It starts with the lung meridian traveling down the arm to the hand, up the large intestine meridian from the hand to the face and the stomach meridian traveling from the face down to the foot, continuing up, down, up, down.

Polarized Universe

Yin and Yang demonstrate that we live in a polarized universe, of negative and positive energy. Electricity is one manifestation of this polarized energy. The negative and positive poles of electricity cannot be equated with good or bad, they are what they are, poles of energy. We are not always as astute in our perception of other manifestations of polarity. Due to *be-mi;* body, ego, mind and identity, many of these polarized expressions are identified as good or bad. This is a mental construct. Living in a relative universe, we all see the world individually, as we see it.

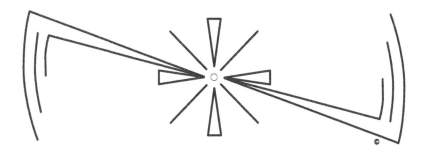

Human body meridians

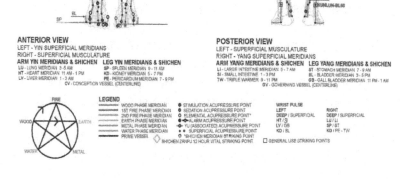

ANTERIOR VIEW
LEFT - YIN SUPERFICIAL MERIDIANS
RIGHT - SUPERFICIAL MUSCULATURE

POSTERIOR VIEW
LEFT - SUPERFICIAL MUSCULATURE
RIGHT - YANG SUPERFICIAL MERIDIANS

Fig. 37

ACUPUNCTURE MERIDIAN CHART

Each of us, at any given moment, perceives our world and existence as fully as we are able. *Pure* perception is neutral. Looking at an object, the visual cortex interprets the data and identifies what it is. Looking at the same object, how you see it may be different. Although this difference may exist, it usually has no bearing on the fact that the visual cortex will interpret the data and identify the object the same for everyone. We can all interact with or talk about the object, with the mutual confidence, that it is the same object. The term, *pure*, refers to the utilization of our five senses, as well as any other perceptual mechanism, without the filter of *be-mi*. Normally, a filter is identified as a tool to clean or purify. In this case the filter is working in reverse. The filter of *be-mi* layers both emotional charges and mental judgments on the perception. Rather than improving or increasing perception, these layers adulterate it.

As charged emotions and judgments *form*, they are projected either toward self or non-self. These projections cause a torque or twisting of the fascial membrane. The result of this torque is a disruption or blocking of *Chi* naturally flowing through *fascia*. This causes an imbalance in the distribution and exchange of *Chi* flowing, as positive and negative energy currents.

As this imbalance occurs, it induces physical, emotional, mental, subconscious or spiritual symptoms. These symptoms are the mechanism that body *fascia* uses to alert us that an imbalance is both present and active. The ability of *fascia to* be the medium for this alert function, is directly proportional to its linkage to itself, which is virtually everywhere in the body.

More significantly, this function comes as a result of the linkage of body *fascia* with all fascial membrane manifestations throughout the physical universe, as well as all non-physical, *pure* energy membranes. Inherent in its very nature, physical *fascia,* is energetically and vibrationally connected to the primordial last membrane separating the *un-manifest, no-thing* realm, with the manifest realm of physical dimensionality.

That which is *source, transcendent* and divine, emanates its spirit essence as sound, through the membrane dividing the *un-manifest* leading to the manifest, to create and sustain all physical dimensions. Body *fascia* is directly linked to the *transcendent.* It's alert system is a direct manifestation of divine grace or guidance. This awareness brings a clarity of understanding that symptoms generated as a consequence of fascial twisting are actually divine gifts. These gifts are like reflections, showing images that can only be seen or perceived through a mirror. *Fascia* is the reflection for *transcendence.*

Symptoms are the reflections only seen, perceived and actualized through *fascia.* Symptoms focus attention. This focusing of attention, induced by symptoms, is a link that offers a window to frame symptoms in *context.* Symptoms are a reflection. Reflections are not the *source.* Reflections point back to *source. Attention* focused on symptoms has precision and intensity. Realizing the symptom is only a reflection, intended to be a portal for consciousness to identify the *source* of the reflection. Source is causality and causality *is source.*

If the alert system is ignored, imbalances are re-enforced as, *be-mi* is allowed to function in an override control mode. When the alert system is operating through a self-realized consciousness, awareness passes through the reflection to *source* as the precision and intensity of focus is relaxed. This is called soft or *oblique focus*. This is placing attention, not on a central area with a sharp focus that increases visual clarity but placing attention at the edge of the visual field. With attention on the edge, visual acuity is reduced while perception and awareness is enhanced. Relax focus, without projecting, trust, accept, let go and let God.

A Physical Blow to Torque *Fascia*

A physical blow to the body, as in a fist to the belly, can be visualized in slow motion. The skin and underlying abdominal organs are compressed. There is rapid forced exhalation of breath, in folding of the upper and lower torso, bulging of the eyes, and pain radiating from the point of impact, like a wave throughout the body. *Fascia* surrounding all muscles and organs twists in direct response to any physical injury.

Imprinting-*Engram*-Fixation Pattern

As the slow motion visual continues, the fist pulls back from the abdomen, releasing and unwinding *fascia* to its original state. What if the physical blow is so severe as to rupture muscles or organs or break bones? Under these circumstances, even after the fist is removed, some level of tissue damage has been inflicted. This tissue damage forms scars and reduces function.

At a specific site of tissue damage *fascia* is distorted or deformed, disrupting *Chi* flow and balance. The distortion can be identified as an imprint imposed on *fascia* from the physical injury. The distorted fascial imprint complex is thicker, tougher, more rigid and less pliable or flexible than healthy, normal *fascia* and tissue. The imprint, is a fixation pattern, which is an *engram.* The example above describes a physical *engram* derived exclusively from a physical source.

When a negative emotional charge or mentally projected judgment, is linked with any experience, memory or image; past, present or future, fascial torsion increases and the imprint or *engram* is magnified.

Using the same physical blow example, what happens when the blow leaves no residual physical damage or imbalance? The image sequence associated with it, or any memory, can be replayed at will. Memory in this situation is a two edged sword. Remembering an experience without linking a negative emotional charge or mental judgment, makes the memory of the experience harmless. This is holding the memory in a neutral space. As a neutral observer, neither the experience nor its memory, exerts any influence or control over us. We are effectively *detached* and operating as *cause.*

The memory of a physical injury, with no residual physical damage, that still has a negative emotional charge linked to it, is harmful. The negative emotional charge twists physical *fascia*, which in turn continues to propagate an energy imbalance inducing symptoms. This is a physical *engram* potentiated from an emotional source.

When the same memory is linked to mental judgment, the physical *engram* is now potentiated from a mental source. Any combination of physical injury, emotional trauma and mental judgment linked with any experience, memory or image; past, present or future, induce fascial torque, forming *engrams* that influence or control us.

This influence is in direct proportion to the degree of our attachment to our self perpetuated *engrams,* causing us to operate as effect.

What happens when a physical injury, causing permanent damage relating to *form* or function, no longer has any linked emotional and mental *engrams*? In this situation, there is a residual physical *engram* still present and damage to *form* and function remain. The physical *engram* is residual, it exerts no influence or control over us because even though damage remains the linkage of emotional charge and mental judgment are extinguished. We are operating as *cause.*

This may seem confusing, since on observation, permanent body damage is present. It naturally follows that this damage is exerting influence and control or limits on our physical or mental capacities. This is absolutely true from one level of perception or awareness. Paradoxically, this truth is not absolute at all levels of awareness. As consciousness expands, we wake up to a more encompassing awareness. The key is found in *manifestation mechanics* that lead to *being cause* not effect. *Being cause* has no direct relationship with the functional capacity of a body *form.*

As the ability to be *detached* and hold the memory, image, experience or projection in a neutral space is actualized, the physical or mental limits imposed by an injury become harmless and powerless to control or manipulate any perceptual, awareness levels, other than the physical. Although a physical or mental limitation may exist, it is only when such a limit has a negative emotional charge and or a mental projection judgment attached to it that we become effect.

Being conditional or attached is what binds us. It is neither the thing, person, circumstance, place nor outcome that binds or limits us. It is how we are, as a function of the *free will* choice of *being* conditioned or reactive versus *being un-conditioned* or not reactive in relation to any person, place or thing that determines whether we are *cause* or effect. Despite the observation of a physical or mental limitation, such a limitation is powerless, harmless and unable to exert any control or manipulate our essence or *soul.* Freedom is a function of consciousness not *form.*

The ability to remember and place experiences firmly in a framework, of being beneficial or harmful, is a critical survival adaptation. There is a potential lesson when a child touches a hot stove that they assimilate and learn not to repeat. Experiences offer a window of opportunity to grow and learn. The lesson learned by the child may be totally functional.

When life experience is filtered through *be-mi;* body, ego, mind and identity the potential to induce more energetic *engrams* is enhanced. The concomitant fascial twisting may generate a cascade of energy imbalances. In the case of the child, will they be able to hold the memory of the experience *unconditionally,* without negative emotions or judgments? This is what is meant when a lesson is referred to as being totally functional.

Experiences are Just Experiences

Experiences are just experiences, neither good nor bad. The way they become good or bad, is how we frame them based on upbringing, experiences and beliefs derived from family, society, culture and religion. These are the pieces that make up *be-mi;* body, ego, mind and identity. Using a cross cultural comparison of severe, intentional body adornment and/or modification, from a common standard Western cultural view versus that of many primitive tribal cultures offers an illustrative example.

There are Nine and Sixty Ways of Constructing Tribal Lays

In Western culture, severe body modifications may be viewed as abhorrent and distasteful. Emphasis is placed on the word severe. In recent decades, there has been a significant increase in acceptance and tolerance of tattoos and piercings in the West. Acceptance of simple or modest body adornment has increased, however, severe body modifications continue to have cultural and social stigma.

In select primitive cultures, severe body adornment and modification is perceived as beautiful. Those that have experienced physical pain to accomplish these ends are perceived as purified. They are honored and held in high esteem by their peers. This is an interesting and diametrically opposed view between cultures. Is one right and one wrong? We live in a relative universe, and as Rudyard Kipling wrote in his poem, *In the Neolithic Age*; *there are nine and sixty ways of constructing tribal lays and every single one of them is right.* (44)

The primary vector inducing body adornment as effect is only when negative emotional charges and/or mental judgments are linked to them, *fascia* is twisted and an *engram* formed.

In Western culture, there are many people that have adorned themselves with varying body modifications, deeply in touch with their tribal nature and heritage, creating none of these energetic *engrams*.

The primitive's memory, from its inception, has neither negative emotional charge nor judgment. Their memory of pain and the presence of the visible body modifications, help them hold a positive image with a positive emotional charge. This memory of a positive image and charge is subjective; it is harmless, unless there is a secondary image or negative emotional charge that develops later that is conditioned or bound with judgment.

As *fascia* unwinds, its edge is released. Subjectively, we experience this release within a spectrum of sensorium that may include extremes of pleasure or pain. The faster and more intense the release, the greater the pain. This pain can be reframed as fascial release, rather than pain that is perceived as harmful. The pain that is intentionally induced with tattooing, to more extreme body modifications in primitive or spiritual circles, is perceived and framed as part of *healing* and awakening. This *process* links into the upward spiral of ever expanding consciousness. It is an active manipulation and releasing of *fascia*.

Limitations of Language

Being conditioned is to be linked with any of five negatively charged emotional states: lust, anger, vanity, greed and attachment. Language is a limited medium of communication. Language is already conditioned.

It uses abstract symbols, subject to interpretation, and has nuances in its spoken *form* like tone and volume and in its non-vocal *form* as body or facial expression, that make its use even more subjective.

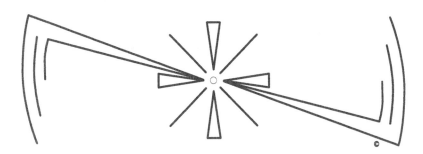

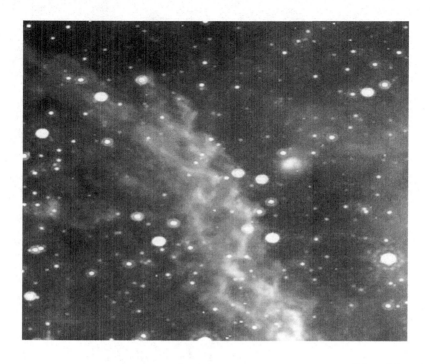

Fig. 38

DNA HELIX NEBULAE

Chi Flows in a Spiraling Double Helix

Chi, or energy, flows through the body in a spiral. This spiral takes the form of a double helix. *Chi* flows up through the feet and out the top of the head. At the same time it flows down through the top of the head and out of the feet. One side of the double helix is moving up as a counter clockwise spiral. The other side of the double helix is moving down as a clockwise spiral. This is occurring simultaneously and continuously.

This helix looks exactly like the DNA helix, although it is non-physical, actuated by sound and seen as light. It is not a coincidence that this helix looks like DNA, because the mirror reflection principle, *as-above - so-below, as-within - so-without,* applies. The above or within is the non-physical double helix, the below or without is physical DNA. The physical DNA molecule is based on the *golden ratio.* (45) It is 34 angstroms long and 21 angstroms wide for each twist of its double helix. These numbers are in the Fibonacci series and have a ratio of 1.1619... very close to Phi at 1.1618...

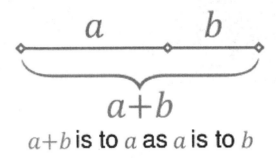

$a+b$ is to a as a is to b

GOLDEN RATIO

*The golden section is a line segment sectioned into two according to the golden ratio. The total length a + b is to the longer segment a as a is to the shorter segment b. In mathematics and the arts, two quantities are in the **golden ratio** if the ratio between the sum of those quantities and the larger one is the same as the ratio between the larger one and the smaller. The golden ratio is an irrational mathematical number approximately 1.6180339887.[1]*

Fig.39

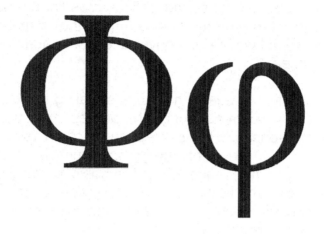

UPPERCASE   LOWERCASE

GREEK LETTER PHI

Mathematician <u>Mark Barr</u> proposed using the first letter in the name of Greek sculptor <u>Phidias</u>, phi, to symbolize the golden ratio. Usually, the lowercase form (φ) is used. Sometimes, the uppercase form (Φ) is used for the <u>reciprocal</u> of the golden ratio, 1/φ.

The <u>golden ratio</u> $\frac{1+\sqrt{5}}{2} \approx 1.618\cdots$ *is expressed in mathematics, art, and architecture.*

Fig.40

The images invoked from the description of the short film, *Powers of Ten* help us to see these mirror image reflections, from the inside-out and the outside-in, they are trans-dimensional. This trans-dimensional quality extends beyond the last border or membrane that defines the most micro to macro-cosmic manifest physical dimensions, to the *un-manifest* dimensions of the *no-thing* realm.

The double helix of sound, reflected as light, emanating from the *no-thing* realm is part of the spirit energy spectrum not visible with physical eyes, or audible with physical ears.

As the ability to see or hear this spiraling helix develops, it may seem as though the perception is with the physical senses. This perception is of an expanded bandwidth of the spirit energy spectrum, beyond the so-called normal range of our five basic primary senses. Whether the result of normal senses augmented or purely extra-sensory, this perception conforms to the label paranormal.

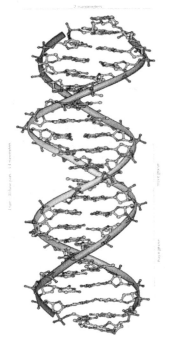

Fig. 41

DNA

Sound as a Portal to Other Dimensions

The force that activates this helix is sound. Physical sound that is audible, is part of a wider spectrum of sound, which as it changes frequency and vibration, becomes inaudible to the human ear while remaining audible to our awakened inner ears. The use of the physical sound, as vocal tones or *mantras,* becomes a resonator that links us to the physically inaudible or super-audible sound. The awakened inner ear is not an organ, it is an expanded perceptual range of sound, independent of any physical apparatus used for hearing. Inherently, the resonant sound generates frequencies of energetic equilibrium to balance physical, emotional, mental and spiritual *well-being.* It also expands consciousness and open portals to other dimensions.

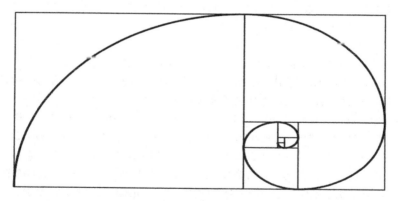

FIBONACCI SPIRAL

A Fibonacci that approximates the golden spiral, using Fibonacci sequence square sizes up to 34. The mathematics of the golden ratio and of the Fibonacci sequence is intimately interconnected. The Fibonacci sequence is: 0, 1, 1, 2, 3, 5, 8, 13, 21, 34, 55, 89, 144, 233, 377, 610, 987....

Fig. 42

The Fibonacci sequence, the Golden Ratio and Phi are intimately interrelated. They occur in mathematics, physics, art, nature and all sacred geometry as well as throughout inner and outer space. This is not coincidental. It is a further reflection of *as-above - so-below* and *as-within - so-without.*

Dr. Royal Rife

Dr. Royal Rife (46) developed a frequency generating machine to treat all diseases, based on the premise that everything vibrates. The concept of vibration is the key differentiating parameter. Every bacterium, fungus, virus and cancer cell has a unique vibratory signature. This signature represents a specific frequency. The correct resonant harmonic vibration, is a specific frequency used to destroy a dangerous microbe or cancer cell. Specific frequencies can also protect cells, organs and systems.

There are many machines that use the concept of vibration to both diagnose and treat disease. Many of the more modern machines are derivatives of Rife technology. A common qualifier used to identify these types of frequency machines is the acronym, *EAV,* which stands for; electro-acupuncture according to Voll. (47) Dr. Reinholdt Voll in the 1950's developed a machine using galvanic skin response at acupuncture points.

Current FDA regulations require that no claims for treating any specific diseases be linked to this technology.

160

Presumably, in Dr. Rife's era, as well as by modern proponents, the contention is that authentic Rife technology may be one of the most important and effective healing therapies ever developed. Current and future research into the applications and efficacy of machine generated frequency medicine is ongoing.

RST, has helped me crystallize my personal reluctance to embrace this machine technology. The definitive answers, both in terms of awareness and healing, come from within ourselves. Externalizing this internal power through symbols or in the *form* of persons, places and things is common and widespread. As long as the choice to utilize an external source or authority, for our *healing* is in *context* and there is no attachment either to it or its outcomes, than this externalization remains functional and is an ally on our awakening journey.

Belief that a specific doctor can, *fix us*, or that traveling to India to find a guru can, *enlighten us*, or that a particular machine, medicine or herb can, *cure us*, is to externalize our own God given internal ability. The power that resides in us is reframed as outside of us. This is taking our divine birthright and projecting it onto an external *form.*

It is important, if or when this choice is made, to recognize and frame it *contextually,* acknowledging it in the most conscious way. Our existence, in the human state, is one in which we are all doing our very best to wake up and embrace our power and self-mastery. This condition is true, even when our consciousness is completely unconscious. It is true whether we know it or not.

We co-create a universe in which we manifest levels or degrees of beauty, wealth, power, love, intelligence, and other attributes. We can place ourselves or view others along this continuum of degrees. Along this continuum we continuously confirm, validate, observe and verify these differences. This ability is a critical step in our awakening journey.

When we frame these observations with a value judgment or negative emotional charge, we torque *fascia* and block *Chi*, binding ourselves in the *Ground Hog Day Loop*. (48) More wealth is not good and less wealth is not bad. Wealth does not automatically bring anyone happiness. We have all observed, heard or read of people whose lives have been compromised due to wealth. We may believe that wealth would never harm us, we can handle it, and therefore, we deserve it.

If we then project an image in our mind's eye of *being* wealthy, we are using the same God given ability, to see ourselves as whole of body, mind, spirit or enlightened. Seeing ourselves as whole, places us on the upward, expanding, awakening spiral of consciousness.

To see ourselves as wealthy, if linked with any negatively charged emotion or judgment, places us on the downward, contracting spiral.

The axiom that *money is the root of all evil*, (49) is a mental construct or projection. This projection is often initiated and supported by family, culture and religion. Money is a *form*. It is neither good nor bad. It is a medium of exchange.

Seeing oneself as wealthy only binds us when we place a value judgment, on the having or not having of it. Linking a negative emotional charge like greed, lust or vanity to the image of wealth binds us as well.

Is it possible to hold an image projection in the mind's eye, linking oneself with wealth? Can this be done without any negative emotional charge or judgment projection being attached to the image? Yes, anything is possible! Functioning as *cause,* the image projection from the mind's eye, without negative emotion or judgment, is released or surrendered to spirit, or the divine. The key, to be *cause,* is non-attachment and total surrender. This is, not my will but divine will, to let go and let God. It is important to recognize that as *cause* we give up our desire or need for any specific outcome. There is no pact between us and *source* that says; if we follow divine direction and guidance, we can ask for or visualize anything we want and the divine should graciously give us whatever it is, because we deserve it.

In the compilation of folk tales and stories gathered in Arabic, the Arabian, *One Thousand and One Nights,* Scheherazade, a character in the book, tells a new story each and every night. *Aladdin's Wonderful Lamp,* tells the story of a magical lamp that is home to a genie. Whoever finds this lamp and rubs it releases the genie, who must grant the holder of the lamp, three wishes. Other than the admonition from the genie that prohibits the wish for unlimited wishes, to kill, or bind another in love, there are virtually no other restrictions. How easy it is to pick unlimited wealth, power, beauty or agelessness.

If wishes are framed through self-will, personal desire and gain derived from *be-mi;* body, ego, mind and identity than due to the universal principles of *cause* and effect, the wishes will backfire as one becomes their effect. This is not to suggest that wishes framed through self-will coupled with *intent, visualization, feeling* and *acknowledgment* of fulfillment in the present moment will not manifest. On the contrary, wishes utilizing this formula are highly likely to manifest. The backfire occurs in direct proportion to the degree of conditionality or attachment linked to wishes that then bind us in the *Ground Hog Day Loop* of *action* and *reaction.*

If wishes are selfless and *unconditioned,* about service to all life, all consciousness, without any expectation of personal reward, they are guided from *source.* Wishes in alignment with, *thy will,* from the divine, are transmitted to and through our essence as *soul,* through our *mind-brain* and body to manifest in *forms* that serve the highest good. The highest good is *transcendent,* it is derived from beyond the duality that allows the mundane, polarized, value judgment derived good and bad to exist. If wishes are framed through *thy will,* then due to the universal principles of *cause* and effect, we become *cause.*

Due to our training as *be-mi,* for most of us, getting out of our own way or our own ego is difficult. If emotional hooks or judgments are present, then the image of wealth we are projecting binds us, rather than freeing us, When there are no emotional hooks or judgments then it doesn't matter whether we have wealth or not.

We are not attached to the outcome. If we're not attached to the outcome and it doesn't matter, than why project any image? Since it doesn't matter, and we have *free will* to imagine and project anything, than why not choose an image of presumed positive benefit, of the highest good for all, being *transcendent?* By *holding the space unconditionally,* we surrender, and allow divine will to manifest, as it will.

One image is as good as another. If this principle is taken as a given, than it is an easy step to decide to project images with outcomes we believe or perceive as beneficial or good rather than harmful or bad. As the laws of manifestation are learned, how to apply, engage and practice their application is critical. Observing outcomes in the long, rather than short term, is one of the keys to personal development and unfoldment. Framing an image projection as beneficial or good has risk only when we link it with an emotional hook or mental judgment. If you *want it,* you *desire it.* Desire is a *form* of attachment. The consequence is that although this power of creative visualization, with intent, can bring us what we *desire*, the desire will bind us in a loop of perpetual effect.

Throw It in the River of Spirit

Take any images, feelings or thoughts, compress them into a tight ball in your mind's eye. Throw the ball into the river of spirit and watch it dissolve. This technique is an act of surrender to spirit or divine will. A great paradox, spirit gives us everything we need, if we surrender and trust. Desires that come from the mind, limit optimal upside potential.

As we awaken, hold a space for needs and wants, to not only be the same, but *unconditionally* divinely guided.

Money is a *form*, a medium of exchange in the physical domain. A primary purpose of existence is to serve life. Can we in our service be vehicles or channels for the use of money guided by spirit? Of course we can, but be mindful and aware of what is known as the *Devils Pact*. (50) Here is an example; *Oh God, let me win the lottery and I promise to use the money to do your will.* This is a bargain rife with complications, probably better off avoided. This book is not about limits, it is about the unlimited. It is about awareness, understanding and discrimination. It is about finding connection and guidance from a non-linear, non-mind, divine *source*.

From the Bible, Matthew 6:24-33 *Seek ye first the Kingdom of God, and his Righteousness, and All these things shall be added unto you.* (51) This kingdom is inside each and every one of us. It is not outside of us. It is reflected outside of us but is actually inside us.

When we understand that the mirror is intended to show us a clear reflection, we have only to stop projecting our own images from *be-mi* to *see*. This is *seeing,* without the filter of the mind obscuring or adulterating the image. Stop projecting or pushing an ego derived warped image at the mirror. Open *soul,* heart and mind *unconditionally. Hold the space to see.* The space to *see* not our fabricated self-image, but the image, reflection of the divine, of God. We suspend preconceived ideas or images that distort true vision. When we *see, what is, it just is*.

One way of expressing our ability *to see,* is the choice *to see soul* to *soul*. We are *soul*, we are not the body. The body is just a shell. The shell may manifest in many and varied *forms*. We may *see*, recognize and differentiate these *forms*, but *soul to soul* we realize, recognize and *see* the *forms* for what they are, merely *forms*. *Soul to soul* the mirror is clear; the reflection, *is, what it is*. Our ability to place value or an emotional charge on the image, person, place or thing defines a limit. This limit obscures the mirror.

We all have an innate natural ability to observe differing levels or degrees, gradations of hot, cold, light, dark, big or small, which reflect properties of polarity, Yin and Yang. This capacity is a critical step in our awakening journey. This capacity for differentiation connected with or without judgment, as well as negative emotions, is what binds or frees us. We are co-creators.

We have created a universe in which, through this capacity for perceptual differentiation, we can choose to see ourselves as more or less than; more or less than someone or something, other than ourselves. This ability to see ourselves as more or less than is not the view of *soul* awakened, it is the view of *soul* awakening.

This stepping stone of awareness induces us to project from the observed lesser space to the observable greater space. When we see ourselves in the lesser space we find it easier to project the greater space on a person, place or thing outside ourselves. This brings us back to the projected image of the doctor, guru, machine or medicine as being the *source* of our *healing* or enlightenment.

As we develop cognitive skills through the identification of ourselves as *be-mi,* our perception is improved through the five primary senses. We perceive, identify and learn the continuum of our attributes relative to qualities or differences like; male, female, tall, short, fat, thin, young, old, sick, healthy and sane, insane.

We have the ability to not only perceive, identify and learn the continuum, we can now also place a value or judgment on what we perceive along the continuum. It is because of the refinement of the five senses and identification as *be-mi* that we have the capability to add a value, charge, emotion or judgment to the attributes we observe along the continuum.

Sick and healthy, sane or insane, are words that are already predesigned to attach judgment as part of their definition. These words, as all words, that can only be understood with judgment as a requisite part of the definition, have a downward and outward energy spiral, they are limiting and disconnecting. If we think, read or speak them we are at risk to be bound in this downward spiral.

As we start to wake up, and realize what we are doing, we may consciously choose to continue to project our inner power onto external objects. From this positive feedback loop, we may manifest in the body or consciousness what we are projecting. As we wake up more we discover that we no longer need to project on anything external to ourselves and that doing so only limits or obscures the mirror.

Do people, places or things have the ability to affect us independent of our own consciousness? This is possible only when we give or imbue power to an external thing, creating a degree of self-induced dependency. We all do this in many aspects of our lives. The key is to make the most conscious, aware choices and fully understand our power and responsibility.

As we wake up in this expanded awareness in relation to our health, *well-being* and consciousness, we may reconsider how much we project our power on anything external to ourselves.

Vibration induced through vocal sound is a powerful and complex internal tool. Is this tool more powerful or effective than an external tool in the *form* of a device or machine ? Any device may be utilized on our behalf.

Be mindful, *unconditional* and observant, to more fully understand the ramifications of choice. If everything comes from the inside out, than the only real power is from within. External manifestation is an external projection from within ourselves made manifest. We give life or power to these external manifestations by acknowledging them. This should be a fully conscious act that does not distract or disrupt us on our awakening journey.

The spiral is moving upward, inward with increasing vibration and frequency or the spiral is moving downward, outward with decreasing vibration and frequency. *Viveka* is a Sanskrit word that translates as right discrimination; the ability to discriminate as to whether we are on the upward or downward spiral.

This discrimination does not frame any experience or condition as better or worse. It is to recognize our direction relative to contraction and expansion. The paradox here is that the upward, inward spiral is expanded, while the downward, outward spiral is contracted.

The *Heisenberg Uncertainty Principle*

In *Quantum physics* the *Heisenberg Uncertainty Principle* (52) states that either we can know the location of a particle or its momentum, but not both simultaneously. The more closely we identify one parameter, the less accurately we identify the other. This gives rise to the particle or wave perception of matter. This is a paradox; reality includes both perceptions, it is always more inclusive and expanded rather than exclusive and contracted. The problem presented, which is a reflection of the *Heisenberg Uncertainty Principle,* is not related to or dependent on the expertise of the experimenter. The problem of defining location and momentum simultaneously, is an inherent part of the natural function of the system.

The *Heisenberg Uncertainty Principle,* represents a clear and unfiltered reflection of our state of consciousness. To paraphrase Paul Twitchell, the modern day founder of *Eckankar* Religion of the Lght and Sound of God; *when we believe or think we know, where we are in terms of our spiritual unfoldment or level of spiritual awareness and development, than that is the one and only time we can be confident, that that is not where we actually are.* (53)

This statement attributed to Paul Twitchell, is a paradox that can be likened to a *Zen koan*, (54) like the sound of one hand clapping, it is a spiritual device to offer a window to step outside the mind and its linear, cognitive *process* to *see* and experience something else. This is a window into a cognitive connection with *source.*

Freeze Frame

The something else, which is *transcendent,* can only be alluded to with language, not understood through language. It is like a particle of physical matter, the qualities of which are illusive to scientific inquiry. A fuller understanding or awareness requires the ability to expand perception beyond the realms of the five senses and the mind. When we believe or perceive that we know exactly where we are in relation to *space-time,* or where our consciousness is in relation to all dimensions, we induce a fixation pattern or *engram.* This can be visually and symbolically represented as a *freeze frame.*

The term *freeze frame* (55) refers to the technique in cinematography where a single image is repeated or superimposed upon itself. The film, *Groundhog Day* is an example of this technique, using the same segments from previous scenes in a sequential series.

This *freeze frame* application, applied to the movie *Groundhog Day,* makes it clear to the viewer that the character played by Bill Murray has been literally frozen in time, as he is forced to replay and re-experience the same day over and over.

Conceptually, the movie does an excellent job in demonstrating how a fixation pattern *engram* of our consciousness, manifests physically. The only significant fictionalization of *process;* the mechanics of consciousness in operation, is the time line of the *freeze frame* sequencing. In the real world the repeating *engram* patterns can range between minutes to lifetimes. In the movie, a single day is seen repeating over and over. This is a brilliant way to attract our *attention* and *awareness* to recognize the essential truth and accuracy of the *Groundhog Day* depiction of the effect of *engrams*.

In the, so-called, real world any experience that we overlay with strong negative emotions or judgments is an experience that we have not been successful in learning the one basic and fundamental lesson that all experiences are for. The lesson is; *all experiences are just experiences, neither good nor bad. The only real power or freedom that can be actualized in relation to any experience is the free will choice to react or not react.*

In *Groundhog Day*, the authentic power of control or change is not manifest as the ability to change anything external that exists in or is part of the world. Authentic change is a change of internal consciousness. This is from the inside-out.

In the real world, repeating *engrams,* manifesting as the same experiences that we are unwilling or unable to release, coupled with strong negative emotions and mental judgments, have a delay interval in the physical dimension with significant time variables.

These time variables can be months, to years, to centuries to millenniums. The more unconscious or unaware of a repeating *engram* experience, the longer the delay. As part of our journey of awakening consciousness, the more aware we are of the *engrams* repeating cycle, the faster and shorter the interval between them until we achieve complete *Vairag* or detachment, at which point the *engram* is extinguished.

Trying to frame where we are, on our spiritual journey, in terms of some type of linear differential, derived from a projected value system that separates levels of awareness ideologically from lowest to highest or worst to best, is like trying to insist that the *Heisenberg Uncertainty Principle* is fundamentally wrong and that we must be able to find a particle's location and its momentum simultaneously. These comparisms are distractions that may interfere or even derail our spiritual *process.*

Exactly where we are, or think we are, on the spiral of consciousness borders on useless and irrelevant. Our direction on the spiral, on the other hand, is useful. We can use it to assess whether we are moving up and expanding or moving down and contracting. As we try to frame this with our mind, using thought or language, if we place value or charge on it, we get caught in the loop. My father always told me; *son you have to choose, you have to decide, you must place value on things, to differentiate right from wrong.* (56) An alternate image as a reframe, either we are in the flow or we are not. More precisely either we are moving up the spiral or we are moving down.

Our natural state, *being* inexorably drawn like a moth to the flame, is to move up the spiral. It isn't good, it merely *is.* We do what we do because we do *it*, we choose *it* because, *it is what it is,* a linkage to *source* and divine guidance. This is not choice or action that is mind based, derived from moral, cultural or religious teaching.

Our ability to frame things and choose from a moral ethical perspective is essential. It is not the view of *Soul Awakened* but rather the view of *Soul Awakening.* From an external viewpoint, it may look to the observer that what we are doing is based on a code of ethics, but if we are truly in the flow, it actually comes from a place deep within us that *transcends be-mi;* body, ego, mind and identity.

When we start to operate our lives in this manner we may initially believe or perceive that some seemingly external force or consciousness is guiding us. As we learn to *objectify awareness,* to *be* the *neutral observer,* we realize the force or consciousness guiding us is *internal.* The link to *transcendent source* is actualized.

God IS too Great for any One Religion

Due to our indoctrination as *be-mi;* body, ego, mind and identity we attempt to frame this experience into a religious construct, based on our lives primary religious exposure. There is a bumper sticker, *God is too great for any one religion.* (57) We have a planet of people that choose to disagree.

174

This disagreement comes from dogma, insecurity and fear. Consider this definition of fear: *False Evidence Appearing Real*. (58) When we realize that we live in a relative universe, how we see the world is how it is. This being equally true for all of us, allows us the opportunity to no longer desire to defend or prove our point of view. We can now afford, each of us, in our own way, to live our lives as we choose and to allow others the same privilege. To be harmonious and tolerant of our self and everyone.

Bruce Lee

Bruce Lee, the martial artist, wrote the screenplay for a movie initially titled, *The Silent Flute*, later renamed, *The Circle of Iron*. (59)

The primary character, a spiritual student played by Jeff Cooper, has apprenticed himself to a blind master, played by David Carradine, of *Kung Fu* (60) fame. He is following the master everywhere trying to understand and emulate his every move. In a specific scene, they approach a river bank. On it there is a hut where a boatman and his wife and family live. They are hard-working, humble, poor people.

The master explains that they need to cross the river but have nothing to pay. The boatman makes it clear that he must receive payment to feed his family. The master suggests that if the boatman lets them use the boat then they will be able to pole to the other side, accomplish their business, and on their return, fill the boat with paying customers.

The boatman agrees, since it is a spiritual master making the request, so surely all will benefit. The student, feeling pride to be with such a great master, takes the pole and poles them to the other side.

On their arrival to the opposite bank, the master immediately punches a hole in the boat, sinking it to the bottom of the river. The student is outraged and demands an explanation from the master. The master proceeds up the opposite bank of the river and off into the woods, offering no explanation to his apprentice. The student follows the master exasperated and angry, insisting on an answer for this cruel and callous action.

The master continues to ignore the student who tries to pick a fight with him. The student accuses the master of being a charlatan and a selfish, mean, spiteful man.

The master continues to blithely ignore the fuming student who eventually goes his own way. This is a critical cusp in the movie. From this point on, the student proceeds to have a series of experiences and misfortunes, while remaining totally disillusioned about the master. Now, with the magic of movies, we shift into a scene where the master has a vision of a band of cut throat thieves coming to the river bank where the boatman would have normally been waiting.

The thieves make the boatman take them across the river to his hut. Once there they force the boatman to watch them rape his wife and daughters, kill his sons, than his wife, than him. They kidnap the daughters and turn them into slaves.

Can we judge the actions of another? Externally, we can observe actions and presume to understand. In the example above, as the observer, we can identify with the spiritual student's point of view, in which it seems clear that what the master has done is wrong.

When we believe our moral compass is above reproach, that our keen insight is flawless and the real truth is our constant companion, that our right to judge is divinely inspired, then our *be-mi;* body, ego, mind and identity has taken control and we are lost.

Imagine the master upon having his vision, moving up the spiral, in the flow, not thinking, judging, projecting or choosing the so-called right action. His actions are not dictated by mind or some relative moral code. The master's actions are a reflex generated through divine guidance. From this *transcendent* space of *being,* in the moment and *unconditional,* the doorway for *source* to guide us is held open. The directive for action or *doing* is an activation of *instinct. Instinct* is a divine connection and guidance that all animals possess. *Instinct* is a knowing, coupled with action, where no thought or opinion is involved. Humans may project or believe that this divine connection and guidance is not available or accessible to them. This is a self-inflicted judgment. Until released, it is as true as any other perception or judgment generated in any polarized, relativistic dimensions.

As the observer, seeing this new expanded scene with all the details filled in, we now have a clearer understanding of the actions the master has taken.

We may now believe, with our still conditioned minds and self-presumed superior ethical training that the actions of the master can now be identified not as bad or wrong but rather as good and righteous. Knowing that our moral compass is clear and true, we, like the student, know our perception, our judgment of the master's actions are correct. We know that the student's perception and judgment linked to his perception was flawed. This flaw was the consequence of insufficient perceptual data to *process* accurately. The student was completely confident he had all the data he needed. In our lofty position as the observers of all, unlike the misguided student, our perception and linked judgment is flawless. This type of ego driven righteousness supports our ability to continue to project judgments and binds us even deeper in its associated *engram* loop.

It seems logical that our previous identification with the student's point of view, which seemed justified, has now been modified, to correctly reflect the truth, based on our having more detailed facts. Previously, we had made an incorrect judgment due to incomplete information. Now we are able to make a correct judgment with complete information. This seems plausible, but what if there was even more information?

What if this new information would cause us to modify our new, current judgment? As we move from the more contracted; the student's level of perception, to the more expanded; the observer's level of perception, it seems that the expanded that is more than is better.

This is a natural developmental *process,* in which perceptually we learn to frame the expanded not just as more than, but better than.

As we awaken, we unfold to even more expanded spaces, eventually moving across the last membrane or edge into the *unconditional* and *un-manifest*, where polarity and duality no longer exist.

In this space where polarity and duality no longer exist, we step across the boundary where language, dependent on duality, is now incapable of using descriptive differentiating terms to identify or relate anything except in the most abstract way. Beyond duality there is no expansion, nor any quality or attribute we may associate with it, such as better than. Framing more, as a projection judgment of better, is a relative truth. Perceiving and framing relative truth is essential, where the expanded is first identified as more, which is linked with the judgment of, better, attached. This is part of the *process* of *soul* awakening. *Transcending* relative truth is essential, where the expanded is framed as more, without linking the projected attribute of better. In the final stage, the expanded is not framed at all. This *is Soul Awakened!*

One of Bruce Lee's trademarks was his use of vocal sound as he engaged in his unique *form* of mixed martial art. Vocal sound increases focal *Chi* intensity. This is one reason Bruce Lee stood out among martial artists. Any martial art or movement meditation that adds vocal sound is essentially a *form* of *RMM:* resonant movement meditation.

Viveka (Right Discrimination)

There are five negatively charged emotional states which bind us and are the basis of our conditionality. To see or understand them fully, in *context,* step outside the framework of judgment.

The ability to judge is derived from our subjective perception of right and wrong. This framing allows us to compare and place a linear, sequential value on everything. Stepping outside the framework of judgment these five negatively charged emotional states can be perceived as manifestations of polarity or energy. Identified as polarized energy states, the attribute of a negative emotional charge is extinguished. We are able to recognize that everything and every experience represent opportunities to grow and wake up. There are no good or bad experiences, just experiences that we choose to react to or not. When we engage any of these five emotional states with negative value laden charge attached, we have made the choice to react.

When we step back and diffuse the reactive cycle we discover that these seemingly bad experiences are as much our allies as any experience. We have developed *Viveka*, (right discrimination), and are now able to differentiate our movement on the upward or the downward spiral.

The five negatively charged emotional states are lust, anger, vanity, greed and attachment. Examining these in more detail, all of them are *forms* of attachment.

All other modifiers or adjectives that describe negatively charged emotional states can be placed as subcategories within these five primary categories.

The Aura=Protective Energy Membrane

The body is encased in a protective energy barrier. It is the aura. This protective barrier is impenetrable from anything outside it pushing inwardly. As long as the barrier is intact, we are unharmable and untouchable. The impenetrable barrier or membrane, however, can be pierced from the inside. To be pierced from the inside-out requires the consciousness inhabiting a particular body to engage in negatively charged emotions and or judgments. We do this when we make the *free will* choice to engage lust, anger, vanity, greed or attachment. With any of these negatively charged emotions we rupture the protective membrane. The resultant hole through the membrane from the inside-out is a portal. Through this portal, from the outside flowing in, the same negatively charged emotion that initially pierced the membrane from the inside-out, can now flow from the outside-in to harm or affect us. The principle of, *like attracts like,* is demonstrated. It is only by using or engaging any of the five primary negatively charged emotions that susceptibility to their influence from an external source can happen. We become the effect of our own causation.

The same *free will* we use to link ourselves with any of these five negatively charged emotions, is the same *free will* that we can choose to find a path to *be cause* and not effect. *Don't project out, don't project back.*

Projecting out is to link negatively charged emotions and or judgments at anyone or anything outside of self. To project back is to link negatively charged emotions and or judgments at oneself. Is it actually possible to be able to refrain from projecting? Commonly, in our self-limiting state of consciousness, we may admit or even insist that the ability to not project is beyond our fragile, weak and inherently flawed condition. This creates a self-imposed limiting barrier that binds and traps us.

No one and nothing exterior to ourselves can free us from this trap. Only we can free ourselves from this trap, from the inside, out. This requires a change in *awareness, attention* and *attitude.* This change is a function of an internal perceptual shift. This shift is derived from a *transcendent* link that allows us to frame our life and all life experiences in *context.* The *context* is the ability to *see* and *be.* That is, to *see* and *be* as essence, as *soul. Soul* is always connected to *source. Soul* existing in both polarized and non-polarized dimensions is able to overlay a non-polarized perception and awareness on anything or any experience or situation. This cuts through the filters imposed by *be-mi;* body, ego, mind and identity. It cuts through the filters imposed by all emotional and mental *engrams.* These filters warp and adulterate perception and awareness. *Soul context* allows us to *see* and *be* with all filters of distortion removed.

Be unconditional, in the moment. Being unconditional is to refrain from putting or placing any conditions or limits on anyone or anything.

To *be unconditional* is to *be* detached. Detached is to not have or hold attachment to any person, place, thing, situation or experience. To not project requires *being unconditional.* To *be in the moment. Being in the moment* is an aspect of detachment. In this state our *attention* and *focus, is here now.* This automatically stops us from linking negative emotions or judgments to the past or future.

To *be grateful for all things, and all experiences.* This gratitude comes from the *context* of *soul.* The awakening or remembering that all things and experiences have only one essential function. This is the function to allow us as *soul* to practice, learn and understand that all experiences are just experiences, neither good nor bad. Experiences offer opportunities to teach us to stop trying to change, manipulate or control the external. These actions bind us in the loop of effect.

Experiences offer us the opportunity to control what really matters. This is our inner *awareness, attitude* and *attention.* To choose to *be unconditional,* to stop the reactive cycle. Ultimately to let go and let God, to just *be.* Is this possible in the physical domain? Not only is it possible, it is a spiritual imperative. The first step is the active engagement of tools like *RST* and *RMM* and then practice, practice, practice.

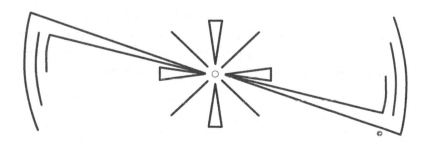

BEING IS the ESSENCE of BEING

LOVE IS the WAY to BE FREE

FLOWING like the WIND

You will SEE

INFINITELY

into the SEA

of ULTIMATE REALITY

As we view people, places, and things we have *free will.* It is essentially up to us how we *see,* interpret or feel. When we are in a reactive mode, we may believe or perceive that our thoughts and feelings are just happening to us and that we are not initiating either. This places us in the condition of the victim. From this perspective, we are unable to control or change. In a reactive mode we are effect. This perception is the result of a lifetime of training and identification as *be-mi;* body, ego, mind and identity. Our destiny is to *be cause* and to control our lives.

Control does not come from utilization of seemingly positive visual projections alone. Control comes from a complex of active and passive *processes,* which lead us through a myriad of layers or membranes.

We contract and expand, finding and moving continuously on the upward spiral until the last barrier membrane is pierced. The control or state of *being cause* that ultimately follows is unlike anything the mind can perceive or conceive.

Plato's Parable of the Cave

In *Plato's Parable of the Cave*, (61) from *The Republic,* imagine *being* in a cave, tied up, looking at the shadows reflected on the wall of the cave in front of us. These shadows are created by the light of a fire behind us. Our bodies are the objects forming the shadows. We are tied so we can only look forward, our total reality is the shadow reflections we see.

This parable mirrors the nature of our perception and consciousness. The shadows represent our physical senses. If these senses are all that we have to perceive with, then any attempt to suggest or prove otherwise will likely be rejected and ridiculed. In Plato's parable, one of the people tied in front of the fire chooses to engage the question, *is life no more than this?*

This introduces the principle of faith, which I define as a state in which we acknowledge the possibility or probability that there is more to life or existence than we know or understand. We are willing to suspend any pre-conceived ideas about what life or existence is and with an open heart, surrender to the universe, anticipating that awareness will follow. Couple this with the commitment to do whatever it takes to find the answers.

With this definition, faith is not a belief in a pre-identified system of dogma that we must accept based on the authority of others, nor is it blind.

Turn the Key of Faith-Open the Door- Walk Through

Religions teach the importance of faith, to which we often cling desperately, due to a simple yet profound need to have meaning in our lives. Faith is a key. It opens a door we are meant to pass through.

In Plato's cave, the individual that has conjectured the possibility of something more to life than shadows, breaks from bondage. Turning around he discovers the fire and its light producing flames. The light is startling and too intense for eyes that have never had to adapt. As the individual examines the fire and looks around, he becomes aware that the fire is the *source* of the light. The fire creates the shadows that are the reflections of his fellow captives. This knowledge is illuminating and expansive.

This awareness does not deny the reality of the shadows, but now places them into a broader more expansive *context*. The attempts of the person, freed from the perceptual confines of the shadows, to impart or convey to any of his fellow captives the reality of his expanded perception, falls upon deaf ears and closed minds. Surely he is crazy, since what he is rambling about doesn't exist. This denial of the possibility of a more expanded perception is in direct proportion to the dogmatic fixation of the other captives to insist that their perceived consensual reality is all there is.

Even though he can explain the procedure, to break the bonds of physical and perceptual confinement, no one will listen, let alone actually try what he is suggesting.

Consensual Validation

Through our five primary senses and our use of language, we reinforce our mutually limited view of our world. This is called *consensual validation.*

Through this *consensual validation* of *be-mi;* body, ego, mind and identity, we create, sustain and maintain our world and our perception of it. It is our comfort zone. We don't want to change. Our comfort zone is what we use for foundational stability.

What we cling to for stability, if it is limited in any way, is actually less stable than an unlimited view. A clear view with clearly defined borders or limits, seems more secure and desirable on the surface. As we wake up, we discover the paradox that a more definitively framed thing or idea, being limited, is not as secure as previously believed.

Returning to Plato's cave, the individual that has awakened to the greater awareness of the relationship between the fire and the shadows, having been denounced, vilified and rejected by his fellows, realizes that he is wasting his time trying to get anyone to listen to or follow him. Walking around the fire, he discovers, behind the fire, the cave continues as a tunnel. He decides he has nothing to lose and although it leads into the darkness, he follows it.

As the darkness envelops him, he has to rely on his *sense of touch* to progress down the tunnel away from the fire. The use of touch is critical as a medium to validate ourselves as a body, as well as demonstrate through the finding and releasing of *fascia*, the membrane through which consciousness passes, that we are not a body. The body is only a shell.

Eventually, he starts to see a small glimmer of light in the distance. As he continues, the light becomes larger and larger, until he approaches the entrance of the cave, where the light is blinding. It takes a long time for him to adjust but eventually he does. As he looks out upon the world, outside the cave, for the first time, the scope and breath of what he sees and hears is overwhelming for his senses and mind to grasp.

Over time, he is eventually able to make sense of this new expanded perception. Invigorated, he decides to return to the cave and his fellow captives where he attempts to explain and describe this new world he has discovered. He receives even more scorn and derision than previously experienced. He perseveres and eventually convinces one of his fellows to turn around to witness the fire, than to venture down the tunnel with him to the outside. Now that he has an ally to confirm the validity of his experience, it becomes easier and easier to encourage others to turn around and follow them out of the cave.

Morphic Resonance

In Rupert Sheldrake's book, *The Hypothesis of a New Science of Life,* (62) he identifies the principle of morphic resonance. An example of this can be demonstrated by observing rats learning a new maze.

The rats are evaluated for errors and the time it takes for them to master the maze. Different rats given the same maze, in a distant location, having no physical contact with the previous rats, will demonstrate less errors and a shortened time interval to solve it. There is a direct correlation between the number of rats learning a task in one location and the speed at which other rats in distant locations learn the task. The larger the numbers of rats in location one, the faster the learning in location two.

In these studies neither original nor subsequent rats ever have any physical contact or communication between labs. How then is this ability being transmitted? The concept of morphic fields suggests that there is an energy field that interconnects and influences everything. Imagine a completely calm pool of water. When a pebble is dropped into the pool, it sends a wave of concentric circles from the center of the point of impact of the pebble, out to the periphery of the pool.

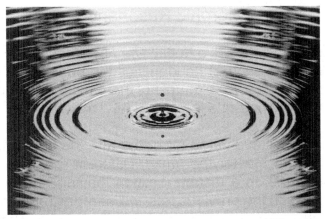

Fig. 43

CONCENTRIC RINGS CAUSED BY PEBBLE DROPPED IN WATER

When these waves hit the peripheral edge or membrane they reverse direction and now act as an interference wave against the originating wave.

If a second pebble is dropped into the pool it induces a complex series of interference waves overlapping and traveling back and forth from the center to the periphery and from the periphery to the center. Imagine the pool as a physical *form* or symbol of the morphic field, an energy field that everyone and everything is constantly afloat in. The interference patterns are induced by our *thoughts, feelings* and *actions*. Everything affects everything else. There are billions of interference patterns criss-crossing, continuously. When these interference patterns are *resonant*, they induce a *harmonic* that transmits across *space-time*.

190

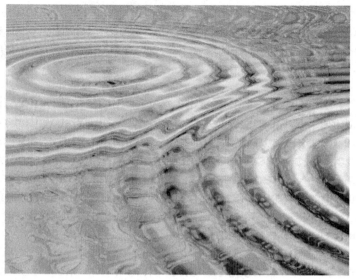

Fig. 44

TWO WAVES OF CRISS-CROSSING
INTERFERENCE PATTERNS IN WATER

Hundredth Monkey Effect

Lyall Watson in 1979 wrote *Lifetide*. (63) He described the observation of Japanese primatologists observing macaques, (a type of monkey), on the island of Koshima in 1952. The macaques demonstrated a sweet potato washing behavior that was passed on from monkey to monkey by observation, repetition and mimicry.

Watson claimed that when a critical number of monkeys exhibited this new behavior, the behavior instantly spread to monkeys on adjacent islands. This phenomenon he dubbed the *Hundredth Monkey Effect.*

Although the actual specific incident in 1952 cannot be corroborated through scientific literature, the concept was popularized by Ken Keyes in his book, *The Hundredth Monkey. (64)*

The basic premise that there is an energy matrix that induces a morphic field which we all exist within and are connected to, has been extrapolated through philosophy, science and religion, all of which are reconcilable, the paradox revealed. The final confirmation is through awakening, expanding consciousness which is understandable and consistently reproducible on an individual experiential basis.

The consciousness we awaken is more expansive and whole than the mind, however, the mind is a useful tool. For many of us the mind is in control and is in a dominant position. This has been expressed as *the tail wagging the dog.*

If we harness the mind as an ally in our journey of awaking, so *the dog wags the tail*, then our ability to use *Viveka*; right discrimination is refined. A body of growing scientific investigation is demonstrating this phenomenon of connectivity. The explanation that this is due to morphic resonant fields is a hypothesis. It is a theory or rational conjecture with an increasing body of evidence to support it.

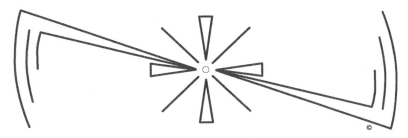

Elizabeth Keyes-*Toning*

In Laurel Elizabeth Keyes seminal book, *Toning the Creative Power of the Voice,* written in 1973, she quotes Alfred Korzybski, known as the father of general semantics, as saying; *the cortex of our brain, is like a large wart or corn that has formed over the thalamic stem, due to the pressures and irritations of civilization.* (65) A significant amount of the cortex can be destroyed and there is not only the possibility of survival but normal function. The cortex is the repository of *be-mi;* body, ego, mind and identity. The brain is a complex biological computer that can be likened to a machine. Garbage in, garbage out, the cortex is only as useful as the programming put into it. The brain is not the root *source* of consciousness. Consciousness exists completely independently from the brain.

This statement revisits the conceptualization of the *mind-brain*. The brain is a biological organ, consciousness uses the brain as a medium for input and output. The mind is not biological, it is energetic and also uses the brain as a medium of input and output. Consciousness uses the mind the same way it uses the brain. Both the mind and brain function as filters of consciousness. These filters do not enhance or improve consciousness but reduce and diminish it.

Keyes writes about *toning* with striking similarity to much of the language I use in describing *RST*. She says, *the idea of toning is not a theory that I am trying to prove. It is a result I have observed... Toning is an ancient method of healing...*

It does not depend upon faith, or belief in the method, any more than these are necessary to our use of electricity to provide light and energy in our daily living. There appears to be certain natural flows of energy in our bodies and if we recognize them and cooperate with them, they benefit us. (66)

Keyes makes a reference to *glossolalia*, speaking in tongues, and compares it to *toning*. When I first started doing *RST* I also observed this relationship. Keyes quotes Marcus Bach from his book, *The Inner Ecstasy; before the coming of churches and temples, before men were certain about the object of their worship, an inner awareness of something higher and greater than themselves filled their hearts with rapture and their tongues with praise.* (67)

Glossolalia is a form of vocalization that resembles spoken language, due to the utilization of inflection and syntax. It often manifests as a series of incoherent, seemingly unintelligible syllables. Its practitioner proponents generally believe it to be a sacred language. In modern Western culture, it is a foundational component for Pentecostal and Charismatic Christianity.

These religious orders perceive it as a message from, or a prayer to God. *Glossolalia* has ancient biblical reference and a heritage spanning many other religious traditions from Africa, Borneo, India, South America, Indonesia, Russia, China and Japan. It is found in Paganism, Shamanism, Mediumistic Religions, Spiritism, Hinduism and Voodoo.

An aspect of *glossolalia* is, *interpretation of tongues.* This is where either the individual speaking in tongues, or someone else listening, is able to translate or interpret the meaning for oneself or others. *Xenoglossy,* is the speaking in tongues of an actual language, unknown to the speaker. This specific phenomenon is identified biblically but in modern times its evidence seems primarily anecdotal, as independent reliable third party verification is little to none.

Singing in the spirit, is *glossolalia* in a musical rather than spoken form. This is a closer approximation to what Keyes calls *toning* and I call *RST.*

There is a *form* of wordless vocal improvisational jazz singing called *Scat* that connects into this spirit, sound, and energy stream. Ella Fitzgerald was one of the preeminent masters of this vocal *form*. Different musical *forms* when emulated through vocal expression represent different *dialects* of *USL;* universal sound language. I have coined the term *USL* to identify vocal sound expressions that utilize syllables of this most ancient of all languages. Some of these syllables are recognizable as known or common *mantras,* others are not. Every musical style or *form* is a *dialect* of the underlying foundational language inherent in all music. All music is tonal, it is inherently part of *USL.* Music generated from any *source*, whether acoustic, amplified instruments or electronically synthesized is *USL.* Vocally generated music, as pure tones is organic and has the highest natural *resonant* affinity link into *USL.*

Non-vocal and vocal music combined generate a feedback loop that either enhances or diminishes *resonant harmonic* links to *USL*. *RST* helps to enhance and potentiate this linkage.

A *dialect* is derived when a group modifies their primary language to create a variant of that specific language, uniquely characteristic to them. This is most often a regional speech pattern and may be influenced by ethnicity, social or economic factors. One of the exercises I practice is matching vocal *dialect* to its specific music *form* or genre. Using *Scat,* as a generic term to identify vocalization linked with specific musical *forms*, identifies different *Scat dialects. Scat,* overdubbed on different musical dialects like jazz, rock, blue grass, classical, *EDM;* electronic dance music, country or blues naturally takes on the characteristics of the specific musical genre.

Glossolalia has a wide range of expression. Those speaking in tongues may be consciously linked to a *transcendent source* with deep awareness and understanding. At the other end of the spectrum, they may appear to be possessed, exhibiting a loss of control of body and voice. This experience is usually followed by little or no deeper awareness or understanding, other than the faith based belief of having been divinely touched.

In *RST* and *toning* there is a surrender to something deep within ourselves. It brings an experience of an uplifting feeling, connection, increased awareness and control.

The energy stream washes through the body reintegrating the physical and super-physical into *harmonic balance*. An inevitable consequence of this is *healing* that extends throughout the body, emotions, mind and spirit.

Love or Power

While attending the University of Alaska, I experienced an upwelling of sound coming from my body. It was my own voice, but as it emanated from me, I was aware of another presence.

At first, my mind wanted to frame this presence as a separate consciousness that was using me. As I surrendered, I realized that it was not separate; specifically, it was what I frame as my higher self; essence or *soul*. It was amazing, powerful and I felt a deep connection to everything. It was like an awakening or remembering. This wasn't new, it was *déjà vu*.

Everything was surrounded by a series of colored bands of perfect uniformity that I assumed was the aura. I was seeing an image that seemed super-imposed on all physical objects. Due to the fact that there were no holes, dark spots or visual anomalies I framed this visual phenomenon, as a blueprint. A blueprint is usually a two dimensional graphic representation of an object broken down into all its constituent parts. From a blueprint an object can be built.

A blueprint is a perfect and flawless representation of an object. A physical object made from a blueprint will never be perfect or flawless. Our essence as *soul* is a blueprint.

The blueprint that is *soul* is neither a symbol nor a representation, it exists. This existence is not the body *form*.

It is *soul* that creates, animates and controls the *mind-brain* and body. For the majority of *Hu*-mans this normal and natural over ride control has been usurped by the *mind-brain*. Consequently, we identify or become *be-mi;* body, ego, mind and identity, twisting *fascia,* blocking *Chi,* inducing *engrams,* manifesting symptoms and *dis-eases.*

Like being poked with a sharp object, the energy disruption and consequent imbalances that induce symptoms and circumstances that are unpleasant and uncomfortable, is an awareness focusing mechanism utilized by *soul* to get us to pay attention. By *being* mindful, we are gifted the opportunity to frame our symptoms or experiences in *context*. Now we can embrace our gratitude and choose to take action steps, not to try to manipulate or change external things but to change our internal awareness and perception. This internal change is an alignment with detachment, acceptance, tolerance and *being unconditional*. It is trust in divine will with absolute surrender.

Returning to my dorm room experience... The sound came from deep inside of me. I felt waves of calm, serenity and balance. I felt *unconditional* with a profound sense of tolerance and love for all things. In this divine space, two people attempted to enter my dorm room. As they started to move forward, it was as if they were pressing into the surface of an inflated balloon.

The tension on the surface of this energetic balloon membrane tightened and caused both of them to bounce back. They were unable to enter my room. The edge of this energy membrane was coming out of me, and I instantly knew that it was the result of the sound emanating from my voice. I realized that the two people that had tried to enter my space were projecting a wave of energy that was incompatible with my energy. It was like two pieces of music that are dissonant. The dissonance is not good or bad, merely incompatible from a *harmonic* standpoint.

In this deep state of reverence and *unconditional* love I was not projecting anything conditional.

The idea that we are unharmable, from any external force, unless we pierce the protective energy bubble from the inside out by projecting a conditioned or charged emotional state or judgment, was coming into focus for me. Our natural state, in which this protective energy membrane is intact, was operating at that moment making It Impossible for either of these people to enter my room.

When we hold ourselves in this *unconditional* space, although we can recognize the experience as a manifestation of balancing polarized energy, we cannot engage *be-mi;* body, ego, mind and identity, placing a charge or value on the experience in terms of good or bad. If we do place a charge or value on the experience, it collapses and dissipates immediately. What dissipates is the expanded perception and awareness that is a natural consequence of *being* in an *unconditional* space.

I realized that this was a powerful energy stream coming from deep within, and like the sound itself, seemed to be part of me, yet distinct and separate.

We frame experiences from the totality of ourselves, manifesting as *be-mi;* body, ego, mind and identity. The framing formed by *be-mi* is a box, which by definition defines a limited space or degree of consciousness.

As we unfold, we often find ourselves in a new larger limited box or space. It is a natural *process* to progress through these membrane boxes, each one more and more expansive or inclusive. What happens when we have an experience, outside any box, outside *be-mi*?

During this experience, time collapsed. A massive amount of information was passing through me. I was offered a choice between love and power. My mind wanted to frame this as a choice being offered from my spiritual guides. I knew that all I wanted was love. I assumed, that since this sound emanating from within me was unmistakably powerful, that my choice for love was a choice that mandated I deny and reject this sound power. Although this experience was *transcendent,* as I was experiencing it I was unable to remain in an *unconditional* space. Consequently my mind was able to usurp the experience turning it over to my *be-mi.* It was a test, a spiritual test. To use power is to lose power.

To use power for the self or to project an outcome on another framed in good or bad, ultimately is to lose it.

I was confident I had it right, or more accurately my mind, having taken its traditional override control position, was confident it had it right. The conclusion at that time was stop, cease and desist. Be a good boy and neither engage, activate or speak of this again.

We are all connected in a morphic field; a *Chi* energy matrix of living spiritual force, manifesting as light and sound. It is a great ocean of pure energy and love. Like any ocean, it has a wave; a pulse that pours out of itself creating, sustaining, maintaining all things through all *space-time*. Like the ripples caused by a pebble, when it hits the edge of a pool, the edge being a reflection of the physical dimension, they return back from whence they came, back to the *source*.

Chakras and Meridians

Energy flows both in and out of the body in a spiral. The spiral is light, activated by sound, in a shape that mirrors the double helix of DNA.

It flows through the top of our heads, all the acupuncture meridians and all the *chakras* out the bottom of our feet into the earth, *Gaia* (68) our mother, creator, provider, sustainer, living, conscious planet. We must place our feet upon her every day. We must *ground* ourselves, connect and receive her energy back; the double helix of spinning light sound, up through the Earth, the bottom of our feet, acupuncture meridians and *chakras* out the top of our heads, back and forth, back and forth continuously.

The *chakras* are a series of spiraling energy vortices connected to the acupuncture meridians. They are embedded and intimately interlaced within the *fascia* of the physical body.

The fact that the meridians and *chakras* are embedded in *fascia* is part of what makes *fascia* such an important structure in the physical body. The meridians and *chakras* previously identified as invisible, non-physical channels, through which *Chi* life force flows, are now both visible and physical as a direct consequence of being embedded in *fascia,* which although thin and transparent, is itself visible and physical. As *fascia* is twisted, this transparent membrane compromises *Chi* flowing through the *chakras* and meridians, causing a blockage or disruption leading to imbalances, symptoms and diseases.

The relationship between *fascia*, meridians and *chakras* explains how and why acupuncture works. Acupuncture needles are used to pierce the fascial membrane at points of increased torque. The spinning of the needles activates the energy vortex that starts releasing and unwinding *fascia* to allow *Chi* to flow unrestricted. As the *chakras* are unwound and activated, they have a direct influence on every aspect of the body and consciousness.

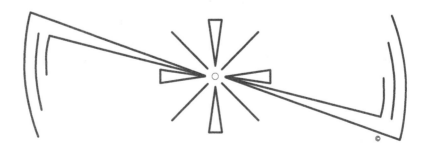

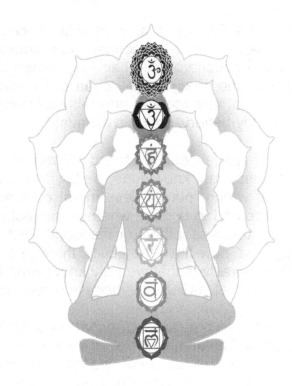

Fig. 45

CHAKRAS

Energy is to flow through us unrestricted, undirected and *unconditionally*. This occurs as we identify and *resonate* with *source,* a surrender to, *thy will.* This is divine will and not self or personal will. The morphic field, being an ocean of energy, is a battery. This ocean, in its capacity as a battery, is an unlimited reservoir of life force. We are meant to be channels or vehicles for it. If we let it flow through us, without directed intent, it is limitless. When we direct it in a specific way, we are cut off from *source.*

We still have a substantial amount of life force energy within us even when we disconnect from *source.* Our bodies are like rechargeable batteries. When we disconnect from the charger, the ocean of life force, we continue to run, operate and inevitably discharge our individual body battery, until it is exhausted.

With our self-proclaimed, new found awareness, higher standard of spiritual knowledge, better discrimination of right and wrong, our flawless moral compass, we are now prepared to engage whatever projections we choose for ourselves, others or the world. With a little knowledge, we now have the ability, through our ego, to convince ourselves that we truly know what is best not only for ourselves but everybody and then act on it.

Remember the axiom, *be careful what you wish for, you may just get it.* The admonition is an awareness that *for every action there is an equal and opposite reaction, Newton's third law of motion or classical mechanics, known as the law of reciprocal actions.* This principle applies to all levels in which duality exists; physical, emotional, mental and subconscious. This is a critical key. We are only subject to the above admonition when we create an image with specific intent coupled with an emotional charge or judgment.

We can project anything we want. The key is to let it go, to surrender the image with no attachment as to the outcome. When we think we want something, the challenge is we want it, that's why we are thinking of it. How do we create an image of something we want and not be attached to it? This is the inherent risk in the indulgence of specific images.

I choose to see myself and others *unconditionally* with gratitude, in harmony and balance, content, fulfilled and in joy. I see this without image specificity. I do not envision a specific job, relationship, house or car but rather the image of a person or situation embodying the above attributes with a neutral non-directed intent, allowing divine will beyond the constraints of right, wrong, good or bad. I call this *HOLDING* the *SPACE*.

Holding this *unconditional* space, allows for the unlimited, for the divine matrix to fill the space beyond the limitations of a fixed image. To choose to see everything *as it is*, in the moment and *unconditional*. With gratitude for all things and all experiences. There is no punishment, no right or wrong. Experiences are only lessons; the lesson to choose to *be unconditional*, to stop projecting out, to stop projecting back, to stop reacting. *Everything IS as it is.*

There is nothing to fix or correct. God is omniscient, (all knowing) and omnipresent, (everywhere) with everything in its place. We don't need to try and second guess the divine or tell it what it is doing wrong or has forgotten. What an arrogant, egocentric view. We once believed that planet Earth was the center of the universe and *HU*-mans the greatest of all creations.

We have proven and been humbled by the fact that our planet is not in the center of anything. What of our exalted self-proclaimed place as the greatest of all God's creatures?

Despite the fact that we are not living in the center of the universe, our egocentricity continues to allow us to perceive God made in *OUR* Image. God is given human *form* in many religious ideologies. Many scriptures denounce idolatry. Humans may choose to anthropomorphize God; giving God human traits. Humans claim God made us in his image. When dissected accurately it is the opposite belief that is true. Man has made God in his image. If God exists beyond *space-time*, beyond duality, then IT is not a he or she, unless we are referring to some manifestation of God bound in *space-time*. God, manifesting in a polarized state, being defined by a limit, is less than the God that *IS*. The God that *IS IT*. God that exists and emanates from outside *STEM; space-time,* energy and matter is *un-manifest* and *unconditional,* IT has no *form* nor any other definable attributes derived from the manifest polarized dimensions.

There is a substantial historical literary lineage relating to the concept of living in the now predating Eckhart Tolle's re-popularization of its meaning and purpose. Ram Dass, in his book *Remember Be Here Now* (69) wrote; *where we are is here, the when is now. There is no place to go and nothing to do.*

The past is only a memory. In this moment all we have of the past, despite any protestations about its previous concreteness, is our memory of it. We can bluster about the fact that the past is real and uncontestable. We can demonstrate with pictures, documents and scars, both physical and emotional, how real the past was.

The question as to the reality of the past is not the issue. For the sake of argument, let us concede that the past is absolutely real. Now for the sake of argument, let us concede that in this moment, right here, right now, all we have of it, is our memory of it. Regardless of the past's absolute reality, the only influence it has on us is our reaction to it now. This is the now of the moment. Without this conditioned reactive response, the past holds no power over us. This makes the question of the past's previous reality fundamentally irrelevant.

The future does not exist; it is only a projection of a possibility. Placing ourselves firmly in this moment, we may claim that the future is coming and it will come despite any attempts we make to stop it or deny it. The rationale and logic of this seems irrefutable. Yet, in this moment, this sacred moment, it remains only a projection of a possibility. When we indulge ourselves in projecting specific outcomes in *space-time,* we risk binding ourselves; becoming attached to *be-mi;* body, ego, mind and identity and the belief that we are no more than that.

Love IS the Greatest Power

Returning back again to my dorm room experience, I was offered a choice between love or power. My choice was love. I assumed, back then, that to accept love I had to reject power. I was now shown that my assumption had been incorrect. I had made the assumption that love and power were mutually exclusive.

That love, in its *unconditional form*, is the greatest power was beyond my ability to integrate at that moment, therefore, I made the choice not to engage or develop the sound energy flowing through me. Despite that choice over thirty years ago, I was drawn to become a Naturopathic physician as well as a dedicated, disciplined, spiritual student. As we wake up on the spiritual journey there is a point where we align and integrate all levels of *being*. This is when every aspect of self is guided and directed from *source*, through *soul*. At this juncture *be-mi;* body, ego, mind and identity are no longer in conflict or resistant to essence or *soul* direction.

The pieces were falling into place for me to come full circle. In 2007 I found myself face to face with the same outpouring of sound energy I had experienced some thirty plus years previously. This time, I was informed that I was ready to bring this to the world. I now had the experience, discipline, *Vairag* (detachment), knowledge and skill necessary to actualize *RST* and *RMM.*

Saying no, was no longer an option. My *be-mi;* body, ego, mind and identity had not fully understood what had happened or how to correctly frame the experience from my college years. My capacity for *Viveka* was unrefined and immature. My awareness and understanding now *being* expanded, I was ready for the next step.

To Give Without Expectation of Reward

We have been trained that most answers come from external sources outside ourselves. This perspective and identification automatically creates dependency. Having *free-will* we can choose otherwise. In the dependent model, although we are not autonomous, we tend to believe that our effort and supplication will bring merit and we will be rewarded. An alternate option is to give service without expectation of reward. Learn to be the giver, not the taker. The more you give, the more you get. This is not defined by the narrow parameters of receiving physical things, it is a function of a higher order relating to what we need, which moves us up the spiral of expanding consciousness. Can we place ourselves in a state that is harmonious, content, balanced, fulfilled with joy and *unconditional* love? The principles of *RST* when applied, offer a mechanism toward that goal.

A Malvina Reynolds song called *Magio Pcnny*, (70) gives an insight into this principle.

LOVE IS SOMETHING IF YOU GIVE IT AWAY

GIVE IT AWAY

GIVE IT AWAY

LOVE IS SOMETHING IF YOU GIVE IT AWAY

YOU END UP HAVING MORE

Healing is a place where we get what we need. Not what we desire, or think we need, but what we actually need, reflected by movement up the spiral.

The presumed desire, or intent to be cured, either for oneself or another is a conditioned projection that is linked to attachment. A cure is an artifact that may or may not occur. Fixation on it is derived from *be-mi;* body, ego, mind and identity and the human propensity to imbue more significance to external appearance and body *form* than is warranted.

We are Receivers-Transmitters and Transformers

The body functions as a receiver, transmitter and transformer. Imagine a radio, this device did not exist until the end of the 19th century. Before the radio's invention, its concept would be so abstract that most of us would find it incomprehensible. The idea that sound could be transmitted by a man-made device, through *space and time,* as an invisible wave *form,* across vast physical distances, to be received by another man-made device, would be ludicrous, insane, magical and impossible.

Today, we take radio waves and radio transmission for granted. The average person does not understand it and does not care that they do not understand it. We are content to use it. This is true of innumerable modern devices that we use in daily life. We are living in an accelerating technologically based environment, which is not coincidental.

There is more than one radio band; AM and FM being the two most frequently identified. The AM bandwidth is between 535 kilohertz to 1.7 megahertz. FM is between 88 megahertz and 108 megahertz.

The cumulative range of the electro-magnetic spectrum is between 535 kilohertz and 2300 megahertz including short wave, citizen band, garage door openers, cell phones and deep space radio communications. The delineations as to which part of the frequency band is which, is regulated and licensed by the Federal Communications Commission or FCC. The radio tuning knob has been pre-set to tune into specifically defined bandwidths. To tune into a different bandwidth, turn the switch from the AM to the FM setting. To find a specific station, turn the tuning knob to the exact frequency of that station. We move between classical, rock, jazz, hip hop, as well as numerous other genres. As we change stations, we are not surprised or mystified at how uniquely different the sound or music is.

Audible sound exists in a narrow band width, defined by the capacity or range of the human auditory apparatus. How is it that we can instantly differentiate different types and *forms* of music within the first notes? Looking at sheet music, the same limited notes are used in all *forms* of music.

This is due to the inherent limits of physical instruments to produce notes, as well as the physical auditory capacity to hear them. The ability to identify different types of music has to do with established patterns of notes, as well as tempo and timing.

With these criteria as reference points, through repetition, our mind is able to differentiate specific *forms* or styles of music.

The body is a receiver. Unlike a radio receiver that can only tune in specific limited wave *forms*, humans can pick up an ever expanding variety of wave *forms*. Light although a different wave *form* than sound is activated by the portion of the sound bandwidth emanating from outside *space-time.*

We perceive the portion of the light band that is visible. This visible portion represents a small portion of the total band, represented by all light. Like a radio, the body, as a receiver, has been pre-set to pick up certain wave *forms,* within limited ranges. The ability to function as a receiver is generally thought to be limited to the ranges available through our five primary senses. There is a body of evidence and research that the perception ranges that seem to be defined and limited through our five primary senses, may be expanded.

These additional wave *forms* are not received through our *so-called* normal senses. The fascial membrane plays a significant role in this larger perception, reception field. Most of these expanded wave *forms* are defined within the context of the paranormal. This area has been popularized within the public domain with mainstream TV shows, movies and literature reflecting a new cultural paradigm of increased belief and acceptance. Not long ago, people purporting to have paranormal abilities might have been shunned, ostracized or even physically harmed. Today, these same people might be hailed as models and heroes.

Some scientists claim that any energy bandwidth perception outside our five limited primary senses is imaginary and not evidence based. Current science is starting to refute this. The work of Dr. Gary Schwartz, who wrote the forward to my book and Dr. William Tiller are two of the scientists engaged in cutting edge research on extra-sensory, psychic ability and phenomenon. The average person's belief in all *forms* of paranormal manifestations is steadily rising.

We are transmitters. On the most superficial level we transmit with physical contact as touch and sound using structured language or not. We transmit with the written word. More abstractly, we feel and think. How much of what we feel or think is transmitted in some demonstrable way to others? Feelings and thoughts are things, they represent invisible wave *forms* of specific frequencies that are broadcast and received. Have you ever noticed when you are sitting in your car at a stoplight and you are looking at the back of someone's head, they often turn around and look at you. This is not a coincidence. Rupert Sheldrake's book, *The Sense of Being Stared At,* examines this question from a research perspective. Nor is it a coincidence when you meet someone at a party for the first time and you either have an uncomfortable feeling about them or an immediate sense of attraction.

This goes beyond body language, eye contact, odor and verbal tonality. Like a dog that approaches with tail wagging or barking and snarling, we have these same senses, mediated through instinct. These senses are the result of energy waves and the interference patterns they make.

We can increase our perception of this energy as we wake up and take back conscious control of the fascial membrane. This is a piece of the paradox of control through release.

We are receivers, transmitters and transformers. Life force or *Chi* passing through the body is partly electromagnetic. The more we are able to open channels for this energy, the greater the flow or charge it carries. A transformer determines how much electricity can pass through a system. The transformer acts like a protective buffer for the system. If you try to drive more electricity than the transformer can handle, a fuse is blown. When the fuse blows, the charge is stopped and the system is protected from damage. Without this protective buffer, serious damage could be inflicted.

RST significantly increases *Chi* flow through the body. In our natural state, *Chi* flows unrestricted. We are a conduit. *Chi* is meant to flow through us. We are channels for it. This is a critically important principle. We are not intended to fill ourselves up with *Chi* force and hold it. If we attempt to hold *Chi* without letting it flow through, its charge builds beyond the capacity of our transformers and we blow a circuit or fuse.

When we hold and project a specific image or outcome, we make a box or *form* an energetic membrane. This box is limited. As we make this box or membrane, we seal off the flow of *Chi*. *Chi* in its natural state, flows through us, not to us. *Chi* is the energy source that we use for manifestation. When we are born, we have the potential for unrestricted *Chi* flow. *Fascia* is still permeable to both consciousness and *Chi* or spirit.

Chi is the life force that manifests and sustains all things, in all planes and in all dimensions that are po-larized. As we become *be-mi* we tighten the fascial membrane, close the hole in the top of our head and lock our consciousness into the body shell. We have sealed the membrane by projecting a box which is a limited view of self. Our tank is full. The body is the tank. It is full of *Chi*.

We have the ability to use *Chi* to manifest anything in our lives. The more we project intent linked with im-ages or outcomes in *space-time* the more we manifest boxes or solidified membranes. As we do this, if we are drawing down *Chi* from our limited personal body tank or battery, then life force energy is progressively *being* diminished. If we are completely permeable to *Chi* or life force, allowing it to flow through us without trying to control or direct it, it is an unlimited resource.

To make a thing or object, *string theory*, postulates that we need a membrane. Without the membrane, *nothing* can take *form.* The critical key is to understand that the membrane must be kept permeable. In this manner, *Chi* continues to flow through. No fuses are blown, no dis-ruption of the balance of positive and negative energy flow and no induction of imbalance creating *engr*ams that lead to physical, emotional, mental, subconscious or spiritual symptoms that can become disease.

We can create or project anything. Any image we proj-ect we are placing in front of our mind's eye now. Even if mentally, we add to a specific image, the mental ab-straction of it becoming reality at some future date, the image itself is not inherently linked to time.

The image is timeless, it is linked to now or this moment. This linkage of an image held in the now, places us *in the condition already fulfilled.* Acknowledging and *being,* in the space of the projected image, as already existing, is a critical component of *causation mechanics* or *process* manifestation. If any projected image is linked to a future time line than it is held in front of us like a dangling fish line never to be caught or actualized. To manifest, the image or projection must be perceived as, *here now.*

If the image we hold, the space we hold, has any negative emotional charge, projected judgment or attachment, we block the permeability of *fascia* and draw down life *Chi.* This is a limited tank or battery with limited reserves. If we use it, we create energy imbalances. We may get or manifest what we want or desire, but the cost is an increase in entropy, which is an increase in the rate of the breakdown of the body and its systems.

People use will, drive, motivation and intent, to project and manifest in myriads of *forms.* This power and knowledge can *be* neutral. Instead, we tend to project our *be-mi;* body, ego, mind and identities perception or identification of good or bad on ourselves or others.

There is an abundance of evidence that malevolent people have garnered wealth and power on the backs and bodies of anyone that would defy them. This power and knowledge is neutral. Anyone can use it for any purpose. We have been led to believe through our *be-mi,* derived from our familial, societal, cultural, linguistic, racial upbringing that we know right from wrong.

This perception of right from wrong is framed in a relative *context.* It is not necessarily a universal constant, even though we may believe or project that it is. When our images or projections are drawn from this relative *context,* we bind ourselves in the *Ground Hog Day* loop of effect.

Having *free will*, we can choose to frame our images and projections with *Viveka*. We surrender to divine guidance. From this point, what manifests is a reflection of *source.* Our role as a conduit or *can do it,* is a direct consequence of us stepping out of our own way.

See IT, Feel IT, Know IT, Be IT...let IT go

We are Pieces of the Fractured Hologram Waking Up

Imagine an ocean. This ocean is made up of particles or droplets. Like any ocean it is whole. *That which is whole, is greater than the sum of its parts.* Out of the ocean flows a wave or pulse. The pulse has a rhythm or beat. The pulse is spirit, made of sound and reflected as light as it passes through all polarized dimensions.

The ocean crystallizes into a hologram, as it enters the domain of *space-time,* and then shatters into untold numbers of particles. Each tiny piece of the shattered hologram retains a complete picture of the original hologram and yet *the whole is greater than the sum of its parts.* We are one. We are a unit, particle or droplet from the ocean. We are waking up, we are remembering. The time is NOW.

RST is a Unification *Process* in Action

The sense of feel is the primary sense that first causes us to trap consciousness into the body by solidifying the fascial layer under our skin, around all muscles and body parts. It is through this same sense, using *RST* as a *unification process in action* that we can reverse this solidification, liquefying *fascia*, which returns natural membrane permeability and frees consciousness.

The Fascial Membrane has an Energy Gradient

The membrane is pierced from the inside by engaging one or more of five emotionally charged energy states; lust, anger, greed, vanity and attachment. When we use any of these emotions, it results not only in a torque of the fascial membrane, it changes the energy gradient through the membrane. The same negatively charged emotional energy that changed it by piercing it from the inside-out, must return from the outside-in.

If the membrane is pierced with anger, then anger will flood back in. The only way that we become the effect of anything is through our own causation. To quote Epictetus; *It is neither the actions of a person, nor things that disturb us but rather our view or reaction to them.* (71)

218

The Way

To Be

Impermeable

Is To Be

Completely Permeable

Holding *unconditionally*, makes the membrane completely permeable; everything flows in and out in balance. The energy gradient is in equilibrium. To *be unconditional,* we stop projecting images with negatively charged emotions and or mental judgments out toward external persons, places, things or situations. *Being unconditional* we also stop projections that are directed inwardly toward self. We stop creating images in our mind's eye with specificity, that is, with a particular outcome attached.

Stop projecting out. Do not create an image of anything or anyone outside yourself that projects an outcome with specific details. If there is a vested interest in the outcome, it becomes an attached outcome. Stop projecting back. When you see yourself in your mind's eye, do not project a specific image with a particular outcome linked with a personal vested interest in said outcome, for it to will become attached.

We are prone to engage projected images for ourselves or others. If we are unwilling or unable to refrain from such an activity, or if we are personally convinced that this kind of imagery is good and proper, which is a personal value judgment, still refrain from attaching a personal vested interest in the outcome. The value judgment, as well as the personal vested interest singly or together link such projected images to attachment.

Attachment binds and limits us. When we create an image with clear borders it is framed in a box. We attempt to control the creative *process*, usually from our *be-mi*; body, ego, mind and identity.

We are Conduits, (can do its) for Spirit

Spirit flows through us because we are conduits for it; for its purpose, the divine purpose, not the purpose of the ego or the little self. If we indulge in forming and projecting images than after we make them, let them go, surrender them to spirit, to thy will be done. Take any image, any intent, and after you make it, throw it into the river of spirit. Release the chains of attachment by *being unconditional.* In your mind's eye, trust and acknowledge this concept for the greater good that is for the good of all. This good is *transcendent* and detached or devoid of any conditions.

The *Form* of the Destroyer

At the end of the first *Ghost Busters* (72) movie, the demon tells the *Ghost Busters* team to pick the *form* of the destroyer. Bill Murray's character picks the Stay Puft Marshmallow Man.

In his mind, he thinks he has chosen a benign and harmless imaginary character. Unfortunately, the demon makes a physical, multi-story high Stay Puft Marshmallow Man that is anything but harmless.

If Bill's character had remained *unconditional,* neither projecting out nor back, there would be no membrane template available to fill with the spirit *Chi* matrix for the destroyer to manifest a *form.*

The demon would not have been able to use our co-creative power for its evil ends against us. Instead, Bill's character pierced the protective membrane of *unconditional* consciousness and became the effect of his own causation.

That which pierces the bubble, membrane, aura, from the inside-out, is now the very thing that floods in from the outside-in to harm us.

See yourself, everybody and everything *uncondition-ally.* Embrace gratitude for all life experiences. *Be* in harmony, in balance, content, fulfilled and in joy. Trust that everything is in order and that *no-thing* needs to be changed or fixed. This can be a two edged sword.

Historically, many spiritual seekers that have entered into this awakened consciousness, recognizing that external action to try to change anything, is not only unnecessary but also fundamentally powerless, choose to do nothing. This choice at its extreme, manifests as a hermit living in a cave or a street beggar.

The awakening spiritual *acolyte* or student, realizes that the only significant choice of relevance or power, placing one firmly and clearly on the upward, inward spiral of expanding consciousness, is the control we exert relative to our personal reaction to anyone, anything or any situation. This is a control we are all capable of engaging and is not dependent on whether we are employed, married, educated, financially secure, have a home, car or clothes. As long as the spiritual *acolyte* is able to maintain an *unconditional,* detached state of awareness, in relationship to everything, the pursuit of anything is irrelevant as a factor influencing spiritual awakening into self and God realization.

Is the choice to essentially do nothing a spiritual mandate? Is the divine will, guiding all of us to ultimately do nothing?

The choice to do nothing is a viable and legitimate option, it is not, however, a spiritual mandate for anyone. As essence or *soul* we are particles or droplets from the ocean that is *source.* The ocean is God. The ocean is everywhere, simultaneously throughout all polarized and non-polarized dimensions. Its wave or current is spirit or *Chi.* The ocean *is whole.* As the ocean flows through the membrane dividing the *un-manifest, nothing* realm, its essence as spirit manifests all polarized dimensions.

We share in the attributes of *source,* we are a part of it, but we are not it. This is *the whole being greater than the sum of its parts* actualized. As *soul,* it is our birthright to wake up and remember who and what we are.

Our primary purpose is to return once again from whence we came, back to *source,* to the ocean, to God. It is also our purpose to make this opportunity available to everyone, to function as a channel or conduit for divine will. This is the awareness and commitment to serve all life, all *forms* and all existence.

The manifestation of polarized dimensions brings duality with all the qualities, attributes and characteristics we acknowledge and embrace. These qualities are usually framed as scientific absolute truth. They include such properties as light and dark, hot and cold, man and woman, life and death.

On the surface, it seems reasonable to identify these polarized attributes as *the truth.* Within the boundaries and limits of polarized dimensions, they are *a truth.* As this truth exists in the dimensional box of duality it has clear borders, edges and limits. It is a relative truth, it is contracted, it is less than.

From the expanded perceptual space across the membrane into the *un-manifest, no-thing* realm, looking back into polarity, that which we frame as *the truth* is now recognized as *a truth.* In the *un-manifest, no-thing* realm there is no polarity. In this space, which is *transcendent,* there is no light and dark, hot and cold, man and woman, life and death. Conceptually, the mind is dependent on polarity to function. The mind has no reference or anchor points to believe or perceive that which is beyond duality, beyond *space-time.* Within the *un-manifest, no-thing* realm, truth has no box, no limits and no clear borders.

This is an expanded perspective, it is more than. *That which is expanded does not negate the contracted, it is merely additive.* More than, is not better than less than. More, as better, can only be extrapolated from our *be-mi;* body, ego, mind and identity. It is an inherent part of polarized dimensions.

Spirit, as it crosses the membrane between the *un-manifest* to create the manifest, becomes polarized itself. The term *Chi* as developed and derived through *TCM;* Traditional Chinese Medicine is by definition polarized.

Using the same quote from Annemarie Colbin; *the Yin-Yang principle is a value-free system of classifying universal phenomena into pairs of opposites...They both spring from the Undifferentiated One, or Infinity; together interplaying in various directions, amplitudes and speeds, they cause all visible and invisible phenomena...they do not remain still but continuously change from one into the other, attracting each other when they're most different, repelling each other when they are more alike.* (34) The ocean and spirit, prior to crossing into *space-time* and manifesting as polarized are whole, they are the hologram. They are the undifferentiated one or infinity. As they cross into the manifest and become polarized as *form*, the hologram explodes or shatters. Pure undifferentiated spirit becomes *Chi.*

As *soul,* as pieces of the fractured hologram, each and every one of us holds the image or template of the original undifferentiated hologram, which is *source.*

The divine mandate is for us to make the great journey home and serve others so they may have the same opportunity. *Being unconditional* and detached does not mean doing nothing. We all have dreams, we take action. The key, is to be more fully aware of the *process* so we can take a more balanced and heart centered approach in our lives. We become masters by applying *causation mechanics* as *process* manifestation. This is the *process* of *being cause* and not effect. As *soul,* our *being* is *transcendent.*

We are no longer bound by or within the *space-time* continuum. We live in this moment, the only way to get from here to there is by *placing ourselves in the condition already fulfilled.* The wishing, dreaming or wanting of anything or any condition, will never bring it forward into manifestation. We have to, *see it, feel it, taste it, be it, Now!*

Being Detached is the Most Connected Place

Do not choose tomorrow. Tomorrow never comes, when we live in the now. To *be unconditional*, we reserve or suspend judgment. We stop reacting. We remain detached, which rather than being a disconnected place, is actually the most connected place. In this place, we have compassion, tolerance, acceptance of ourselves, everyone else and everything. This makes the *fascial* membrane completely permeable. Energetic equilibrium is maintained. Physical, emotional, mental and spiritual *well-being* and balance is realized.

Your Reality is a Fantasy and Your Fantasy is Killing Me

Driving to a drumming circle, I turned on the radio and one of my son's CDs started to play. The song lyrics were: *Your Reality is a Fantasy and Your Fantasy is Killing Me. (73)*

Listening to this song, I realized that it was describing the actual reality we have placed ourselves in right now, right here. We need to wake up; to understand when the power we hold has images linked with negative emotions and judgments. We need to teach ourselves, and each other, to recognize images projected in our mind's eye with emotional hooks and or judgments. To recognize and then release the emotions and judgments and practice *being* the *neutral observer.* To authentically reflect these observations for ourselves and each other, and change what empowers us as *cause,* which is not the changing of external things, but our internal *attitude, awareness* and *attention.*

If the majority of humanity, succumb to images with negative emotional charge and judgment that are driving and perpetuating potential negative outcomes, we risk manifesting these outcomes.

Our ability to recognize and identify images we link with negative emotions or judgments, and then effectively neutralize them, is a critical developmental step on our journey of awakening. As we recognize these images, we may attempt to neutralize them by using our minds.

226

With the mind, we can frame these negatively charged images as bad or undesirable. As we frame the negatively charged images as undesirable, we can then project our will or desire for these charged images to go away. An internal dialogue, observation and identification may take this *form*; 'I don't like this image, it feels terrible. My stomach hurts. I can't stop shaking. I ache all over, have no energy and can't concentrate or think straight. I'm going to try my best to ignore and avoid this image and the horrible feelings associated with it.'

Images, whether memories or projections associated with physical, emotional and mental injury or trauma, linked with negative emotions or judgments become *engrams*. An *engram* is an energetic imprint or fixation pattern. It is a self-perpetuating negative feedback loop. When negative emotions remain attached to an image, a mental projection with the intent on that image, of not wanting it, will not affect or modify the outcome. If you are in a cage with a hungry lion and feel fear linked with an image of the lion eating you, you are using your co-creative power to ensure that outcome.

If you continue to feel this fear and maintain the same image of becoming the lion's dinner, while mentally projecting the desire to be left alone and not eaten, you will still be eaten, regardless of your desire. If the unrelenting fear and repeating image of being lion food is released or withdrawn from both the conscious and subconscious mind, then our capacity to be *cause* has been activated. The lion will not eat us, even if still hungry.

This is the space that Daniel held in the biblical story of the lion's den. Daniel's not being eaten is attributed to his absolute trust and faith in God protecting him.

Daniel's trust in the divine allowed him to suspend his fear and not project an image of himself as lion food.

The human capacity to suspend negative emotions and judgments linked to images is often actualized because of a believed or perceived supernormal protection or guidance. What one believes is impossible, now becomes possible, if linked to or augmented by something greater and more powerful than ourselves. Whether one believes in, knows of, or *IS* a conscious part of *source* or the divine, this relationship at any level helps empower us with increased functional capacity. At one level this induces a degree of empowerment, the cautionary caveat, is not to give or surrender too much power or authority to any external source, which induces varying degrees of dependence. Paradoxically absolute, total surrender to the *transcendent,* divine will, *source* is essential. This never causes dependence but rather interdependence. *Viveka,* as highly refined right discrimination, is a prerequisite.

Our first layer, or level of co-creative control, as *cause,* is in our ability to control and choose the feelings we link with images, whether the images are memories or projections of possibilities. Until we can master this emotional level, what we think about any image is powerless to have any effect. An axiom, borrowed from Star Trek is; *resistance is futile.* The desire or thought that some negatively charged image or thing, will not happen to or affect us, will not make it so.

Trying to erase, avoid or deny negative emotionally charged images, induces the *law of reversed effort*. What we see and feel will persist, despite our desire or thought that it will not.

In a possible projected future, the majority of humanity continues to feed and self-perpetuate a loop of negative emotionally charged image outcomes. In this projection, only a minority of people will discover and actualize their total potential. The expanding wave of consciousness necessary to induce critical mass for everyone's self-actualization will be projected into an imaginary future to remain inaccessible to the many. This trend has happened before and might happen again unless, we as individuals, as well as collectively, make a different choice. Here is a way to reframe this possible outcome.

It has been said that many have been called but few will be chosen but *I HOLD the SPACE that all have been called and the time is NOW!* I invite everyone to share and hold this space with me.

The Magnetic Poles are Shifting

In Gregg Braden's, *Awakening to Zero Point*, the zero point he is referring to is the shifting transposition of the Earth's magnetic poles. This geophysical phenomenon is a scientific fact and has happened many times in geophysical history. We are currently in this shift.

While watching a special on the Discovery channel recently, it was explained how in real time on a daily basis, the magnetosphere is being tracked. A mass of North Pole magnetism covering half of the Antarctic continent was displayed. This mass of North Pole magnetism is no longer in flux, it is stable at the South Pole. On the rest of the planet, fluctuating masses of both South and North Pole magnetism were detected all over the surface.

Animals are sensitive to Earth magnetism and migration routes are linked to this sensitivity. The increasing incidence of whales beaching themselves and being found in remote areas, not normally part of their migration patterns, is attributable to this shift in magnetism.

Other anomalous animal behaviors may also be linked to this shift. We are animals too. Are we affected by Earth magnetism? There is a body of evidence to suggest we are. Gregg Braden makes an interesting argument for the idea that the shift that is transposing Earth magnetism, is also flipping polarity within the body.

Yang is Becoming Yin and Yin is Becoming Yang

Oriental Medicine identifies Yin and Yang. These two qualities define the polarity inherent in the physical universe. That which is Yang is expansive, while Yin is contractive. Everything in the physical universe can be identified as expanding or contracting. Imagine polarity completely reversed in a short window of time. Things would probably get a little chaotic, or maybe a lot chaotic.

Imagine that female energy becomes male and vice versa. John Gray's work; *Men are from Mars and Women are from Venus* (74) figuratively supports the premise that the sexes must be from different planets, since we have such difficulty understanding each other. Imagine before we understand each other or anything for that matter that the properties or qualities of people or things become their opposites.

Braden suggests that to the extent that we are fixated and dogmatic in our life and world view, as the planets polarity is reversed, is proportional to the degree to which we will be torn apart physically, emotionally, mentally and spiritually.

The counterpoint is that the more we are *unconditional*; able to be fluid, detached, non-fixated, non-dogmatic, like a willow in the wind, able to bend rather than break, the less the change in magnetic polarity will affect us.

The time is NOW, this is our wake up call. The incidence of psychiatric disorders for all age groups is rising dramatically. Physical ailments, particularly in the auto-immune category, are increasing, causing reactions to food and the environment.

If everything is flipping, then it starts to make sense why the body's immune system would become confused and attack itself.

Inviting the Spirits of the Four Directions

Through utilization of *RST*, I became aware of a data stream of information that was not inherently or obviously my own. I was receiving what my mind wanted to frame as external guidance. This is an interesting paradox. We are all one. We are all pieces of the fractured hologram. Even when we think we receive or perceive a piece of information from a *source* external to ourselves, it is not.

The guidance led me to invite the presence of the spirits of the four directions of the compass: East, West, North and South. I was guided to make this invitation prior to the initiation of any treatment sessions or any sacred activity. When I resisted this guidance, I would consistently get lost. Lost, as in losing my ability to navigate from one physical location to another. An example would be; difficulty finding my way from my home to my office. This was disconcerting and disturbing, yet humbling. I quickly learned to pay attention. It was as if *Gaia*, the conscious planet, was both asking and reminding me to honor our sacred interconnectedness.

During an *RST* session the resonant sound that was coming through me, took on auditory characteristics that resembled chanting from diverse cultures and languages. Vocal patterns that my patients and I have observed and identified include Native American, Oriental, Middle Eastern, East Indian, African and Gaelic. Sometimes during *RST* sessions these vocal patterns spring spontaneously from patients. On multiple occasions, patients during treatments seem to manifest Xenoglossy.

This is the *form* of glossolalia in which an actual language, unknown to the speaker, is spoken.

A noteworthy incident during an *RST* session, manifested when a Christian patient started singing sounds that resembled Hebrew prayers or chants. When this occurred, I stopped the session and inquired if the patient was cognizant of his vocalizing. He volunteered that he was aware that he seemed to be vocalizing a language, unknown to him, in a distinct rhythmic pattern. He thought the language might be Hebrew. I agreed and we both acknowledged that neither of us spoke nor understood any Hebrew, yet felt that this was either a patterned facsimile of it, or the actual language.

In another case, an older gentleman, raised as a Catholic, who had chosen for most of his adult life to reject any religion, professing to be agnostic, during *RST* sessions, would rapidly repeat, in English, obviously Christian prayers.

When this occurred, as in the previous case, I would stop the *RST* session and ask the patient if he was aware of what he was doing? Curiously, in this case the patient had no cognitive perception of this occurring. In fact, he would vehemently deny that he was doing any such thing. Regardless of how often this occurred, or how often I would interrupt the sessions, he was never able to perceive or acknowledge this phenomenon.

What is happening in these situations? My experience is that the *process* of *RST* activates or links either or both the therapist and patient, with varying degrees of awareness or understanding, into a data stream previously unavailable. This connection is a *transcendent* linkage with *source*, offering divine insight and guidance. Does *RST* have a *shamanic* component?

Shamanism (75) has always been a part of the human experience. Its historical, archeological presence is as old as mankind. Indigenous people, as clans or tribes, all over the planet have always had a medicine person, healer or priest to guide, treat and offer insight to maintain clan stability and survival. These individuals have an expanded awareness or knowledge of plants, animals, weather, migration routes, water sources and other variables critical to tribal well-being. The tradition of a medicine person taking and training one or more apprentices to develop proficiency in these areas assured continuity.

Some of the *shamanic* awareness and knowledge comes from paranormal *sources*. Often the medicine person would use ceremony and ritual, as well as *entheogens* (76) to enhance or potentiate inner guidance. *Entheogens* are consciousness expanding sacred plants that make information and *source* guidance more accessible. These plants are initiators into a mystical linkage. *Entheogens* have historically been used as a screening tool to identify apprentices. Those demonstrating the ability to use the *entheogens* to catalyze a *transcendent,* divine link could enter the pool of *acolytes,* from which additional screenings would identify those allowed to remain as true apprentices.

Authentic *shamanism*, although initially catalyzed from an external *source*, ultimately must be caught, not taught. Without the ability to access the internal *transcendent* divine direction and guidance, the seeming *shaman* is hollow and not functioning as the *conduit* they are intended to be. It is that which is *transcendent* and internal that must be caught.

A curious phenomenon, gaining popularity in the West is the interest and study of *shamanism*. Classes and schools being promoted by self-proclaimed *shamans* offer the attendees a certificate or degree so they too can call themselves *shamans*.

This is a classic example of the West adulterating whatever it deems convenient or expedient.

Indulging in this type of training may certainly derive some personal and even valuable awareness. Does a piece of paper make anyone a *shaman?*

Early on as *RST* was being developed, I was *being* guided by spirits and was drawing on many past life experiences as a healer and medicine person. The information and guidance leading me, was from an internal, rather than external source or authority.

Due to my formal training as a Naturopathic physician, discipline in sound *mantra* meditation, and personal cultivation of *Chi*, *RST* has manifested as a balance between science, art, tradition and experimentation.

Our True *Form* is a Sphere

We are not the body. The body is only a shell. If the body is only a shell, then what is our true *form*? If we exist beyond *space-time*, beyond polarity or duality then our *form* is genderless. In the writings of Carlos Castaneda, he describes the body *form* as a luminous egg. In Alex Gray's *Sacred Mirror,* (77) his paintings portray an egg shaped light around the body. Both are seeing the energy shell or matrix connected with or around the body. Since the body is elongated, when one sees or imagines light energy around it, the light is pulled to conform to the body shape. Our essence or shape without the influence of a physical body, is spherical. If our essence is bound by a body, it warps or pulls the spherical *form* to conform to its own physicality.

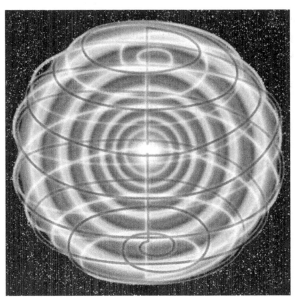

Fig. 46
A SPHERE REPRESENTING THE EDGE
AND BEYOND+COLOR RAYS

Our essence is spherical, our consciousness is at the center of the sphere. From this central vantage point we can focus sharply or diffusely to perceive the distant edge or membrane of the three dimensional sphere in all vertical and horizontal aspects of its 360 degrees, as well as multi-dimensionally.

From the core or center of the sphere radiating out, spirit manifests as *Chi* spiraling clockwise, toward the periphery or edge. This *out-flow* is one side of the double helical *form* of spirit as cosmic universal *Chi* emanating from inner dimensions.

From the periphery or edge of the sphere radiating in, spirit *un-manifests* as *Chi* spiraling counter-clockwise toward the core or center. This *in-flow* is the other side of the double helical *form* of spirit as essential life force *Chi* emanating from Earth. Expand this image to include all the possible combinations and permutations of the directionality of the double helix in relation to the sphere.

Like the parable of the blind men and the elephant, I was shown different angles and perspectives, all of which were right but none of which were comprehensive or totally inclusive. Allowing undirected *Chi* to flow without restriction through a patient, as *fascia* unwinds, the body enters into an equilibrium state, which bursts with bands of all the physical color rays in concentric rings. The physical color rays are seen in rainbows and are represented by the acronym, ROY G BIV; which stands for red, orange, yellow, green, blue, indigo and violet.

This visual manifestation is identical to what I saw and observed the first time this happened in my *dorm room* experience, when I was a sophomore, attending the University of Alaska. This rainbow of concentric color bands is a result of the double helix of spirit, *Chi* hitting the surface of body *fascia* when it is permeable everywhere simultaneously from the *inside-out* and the *outside-in*. This is the *blue-print* or *soul-print* transposing itself on and through all the layers of the physical body, as well as all multi-dimensional energy shells utilized by *soul*. As light hits the surface of a prism it induces the seven primary color rays to pass out the other side. This is analogous to spirit *Chi* as it hits the facial surface, inducing unwinding, leading to fascial permeability.

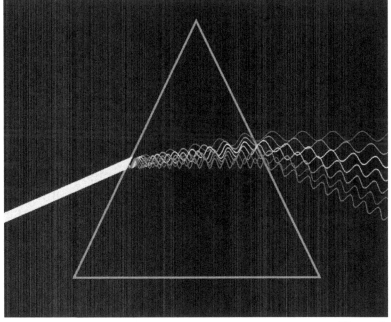

Fig. 47

LIGHT HITTING SURFACE OF PRISM

The phenomenon of spontaneously perceiving color rays around the body is not a projection. It is not intended or desired, it is not induced or imposed upon a patient. It is a neutral observation. This is an observation of the body's energy state in its balanced, normal natural condition.

The presence of the body's color bands manifest, as energetic equilibrium and fascial permeability is established. This happens as a function of surrender and acceptance of divine will and is potentiated with *RST* and *RMM*. The color bands cannot be brought forth with a linkage to a specific intent, to cure or fix anything. If we try to control or manipulate an outcome while the color rays are perceptually present, the image collapses. This is white magic, the projection of a presumed or theoretically positive outcome toward self or others. This is an attempt to control or manipulate spirit. It is an attempt to control God or direct its will from our *be-mi;* body, ego, mind and identity.

The attempt to direct or control spirit will collapse the body's naturally present color bands. Trying to control or direct spirit causes a torque or twist in the fascial membrane. This induces a disruption in the equilibrium of positive and negative energy poles, made manifest as the double helix of *Chi* life force. The energy disruption causes physical, emotional, mental, subconscious and spiritual aberrations that induce *engrams* leading to symptoms and dis-ease.

Let It Be

We are conduits for Spirit, manifesting as energy, or *Chi*, flowing through us. To identify that something is wrong or broken, is an image generated from our mind's eye, as a memory or projection.

Instead of attempting to correct this by changing something externally, or giving the power to someone or something external, we can acknowledge how we co-create, and choose to see and *be* our essence as *soul.* This imbues us with the discrimination to function as *cause* and not effect. In this moment, place the *blue-print,* as the *soul print* superimposed on the physical, emotional, mental, subconscious and spiritual self.

The view point of *soul,* from the center of essence or self, as a sphere, is a 360 degree, multi-dimensional perceptual state. The double helix flows from the core out and from the edge of the membrane in. Perceptual awareness of this pattern of *Chi* flow is neutral. There is no emotional hook or mental projection linked to it. Perception is a perception of *being,* not doing. In our capacity as a conduit, we allow *Chi* to flow through us, without linking a projection of personal will or intent. As a channel for spirit, we allow it to pass through us, to do what it will, trusting with surrender, tolerance and acceptance for any outcome. Spirit, through divine will, brings the *highest good.*

Linguistically, since language is *mind-brain* generated and its structure is based in a polarized framework, how do we use words to express or describe something not polarized? In the case of *chaos,* this is accomplished by describing what it is not, rather than by what it is. The *highest good,* refers to a place or space outside or beyond polarity.

Comparative terminology is polarized; framing things or concepts in a sequential pyramid that designates and differentiates value. Good, better and best are simple adjectives we use to convey this value differential.

Perception, as *soul,* emanates from the center of the sphere; a point in the realm of *no-thing*, that which is *un-manifest. Being* is a state *of* consciousness in this *no-thing* space. As consciousness reaches the membrane dividing the *un-manifest,* moving as an *outflow* into the manifest and passing through the membrane, what does it perceive? This transition introduces the capacity, *to know.* This *knowledge* is bound to and completely dependent on polarity. To *know* a thing, person or concept is to describe or frame it by comparison. Can you describe or identify a thing, or explain anything, without using comparison or relative value?

The biblical description of Adam and Eve in paradise describes how they were seduced by the *serpent* and fell from grace. This was a consequence of eating the apple from the tree of *knowledge.* This is a parable. Adam and Eve, as *soul,* exist beyond polarity. They are genderless. Their existence, is a *pure* state of *being.* They have no *knowledge,* no awareness of duality.

Soul's emergence from the *un-manifest, no-thing,* no time realm into the dimensions of *space-time* and polarity, is neither an accident nor divine punishment. It is a divine gift from *source,* for *IT* to know itself, through manifestation into *form,* using us as the medium of awakening self-awareness.

Source knows itself through the remembering and awakening journey of its particles as *soul,* entering into the dimensions of duality and then returning home to *pure being* with *knowledge* of polarity intact. With this *knowledge, soul* frames itself and its relationship to the divine, using comparison and relative value.

This opens a window for *soul* to frame its existence in polarized dimensions as a transitional step in its awakening journey. Applying the *knowledge* of how to utilize *forms* to catalyze *transcendence* into the *formless,* is a crucial part of the *process* of *soul's* journey home.

Utilizing a two dimensional visual framework, above the membrane that separates the *un-manifest* from the manifest, is the *pure positive.* In this space the only thing that exists is the *highest good.* The *pure positive* just *is,* it cannot be compared or be given value relative to anything. In the same way, the *highest good* just *is* and cannot be compared or be given value relative to anything either. Below the membrane that separates the *un-manifest* from the manifest is the *pure negative.* The *pure negative, being* polarized, is made of both positive and negative charge. When awareness of this duality is neutral, we remain *unconditional,* we are *cause* and control our destiny.

242

When awareness of this duality is linked with negative emotions or mental projection judgments, it is not neutral but reactive. This reactivity is conditional; we are effect and destiny controls us.

Soul's emergence into polarity is not divine punishment but a divine mandate to wake up and take our rightful place as co-workers with the divine. This mandate is for us to master *causation mechanics. Soul's* emergence into polarity comes with an intact divine link to guide us and accelerate our journey home. The divine is neutral, it neither punishes nor rewards. The divine link can only be broken or disconnected by us. Punishment and reward are mental abstract projections generated by our *be-mi;* body, ego, mind and identity. *The only judgment that holds any power over us is our own self creation and self-projection.*

In the parable of Adam and Eve's fall from grace, this fall was not God's will but self-will, derived from the *mind-brain.* The *mind-brain* is the tree of *knowledge,* activated by the self-will act of eating the symbolic apple. As long as consciousness is linked and bound through *be-mi,* our fall from grace is sustained. Our emergence, back from polarity across the membrane into the *un-manifest,* is *soul's* return to paradise; to *source.* The *mind-brain* is a *form*, it is conditional. It controls us as effect only to the extent that we allow it.

To *become formless* and *unconditional*, we must release the hold of the *mind-brain.* In total surrender, our divine link as *soul,* which is *transcendent,* is reestablished. Divine grace, that was never taken away, is found as if anew.

As conduits for divine will, we are *cause* and our destiny is ours to control once again.

Our birthright as *soul* is to *be* a channel; *thy will be done*, not my will or my desire but the will of the divine, the will of the hologram, of the *one*. To quote John Lennon and Paul McCartney, *Let It Be.* (78) From this position we are not invested in the outcome. We can trust. We can just, *Let It Be.*

We are exposed to many and varied external *forms*. They generally come from *be-mi*. They are things or they manifest as familial, social, cultural, political, religious mandates, doctrines and behavior codes.

The *forms* also exist as jobs, sports, games, martial arts and other activities. *RST* and *RMM* are *forms* as well. Their edges or membranes are living, fluid and malleable. They are not defined in a limited box, but rather an expansive one. By definition a *form* must have a membrane. If it has a membrane, then its boundaries are defined; by definition it is limited. Given that we interact with many *forms,* can we use *Viveka,* as right discrimination, to preferentially interact with those *forms* having fluid and permeable membranes? This is *free-will,* the choice is ours, *carpe diem; seize the moment!*

The divine is unlimited. God is unlimited. *Soul* is unlimited. *Forms* are used as a medium for more awareness and understanding. F*orms* are designed as gateways to the *formless* or *transcendent.* We have but to find and utilize the keys to open these gateways, to start our journey home to *source.*

The *Form* is not the Way

The Way is the~~~Way

The *Form* can point, or lead to the~Way

So Master the *Form*, then Release it,

And Remember,

The *Form* is not the Way

The Way is the~~~Way

RST is a *form* and a tool. There are many tools in our tool bag. Recognize them for what they are; tools. Do not get confused or place undue trust or dependence on any of the tools. Optimize the lessons and growth that can be derived from the tools. Ultimately *transcend* all tools. Live in this moment. Do not let the mind confuse you. Open your heart and trust.

The Matrix and *Avatar*

In the movie *The Matrix* (79), the majority of humans in their physical bodies, are being kept in a state of perpetual hibernation induced by a machine dominant intelligence. The machines are using human life force energy as a power source.

Human consciousness is locked into a *virtual reality* artificial world that they are incapable of recognizing as a virtual world. They remain content and complacent with no cognition of their true condition.

The last movie in the *Matrix* series shows that some humans are still living in the real or actual world. In their one safe enclave they celebrate life and freedom. This celebration demonstrates the Earth connected, tribal character of authentic free and conscious humans. This is in direct counterpoint to the virtual world that emulates modern *Western Culture,* incorporating large cities with distracted and disconnected contemporary life.

The celebration of the freedom of consciousness in the real or actual world is powerful and moving. There is drumming, music and dance. The sense of community, tribe and joy are palpable.

The movie, *Avatar* (80) depicts humans on a planet inhabited by seemingly primitive indigenous people. The people from our planet have come for natural resources no longer available on their home world. The indigenous people are *grounded* and tribal. They have a symbiotic relationship with their planet; a living consciousness and all her life *forms*. The beauty, intelligence, simplicity, joy, harmony, peace and contentment of these people is delightful.

Technology has created a machine that can transport human consciousness into a cloned *Avatar* body. This body shell template is in the *form* of the indigenous people. The *Avatar* body is devoid of consciousness until the human connection is made.

Soul, awakened, in balance and harmony, linked with *source,* will manifest a body shell to inhabit, learn and grow from, which is in energetic equilibrium. The human physical body is the cumulative product of our *be-mi;* body, ego, mind and identity. This body is disconnected from *source* and not in energetic equilibrium. In the human body guided and directed from our *be-mi,* we are in a trance.

In the human body *form,* in the world we have manifested through our charged negative emotions and mental projection judgments, we are like the humans trapped in the *virtual world* of the *Matrix.* The fact that it is the *mind-brain* that generates the power in the *Matrix* to run the machines that bind human bodies and consciousness is a modern parallel to Plato's *Parable of the Cave.*

Our birthright, as *soul,* is to find and maintain our link with *source.* We are children of Earth, *Gaia;* she is a living conscious planet Like awakened *Avatar,* we are part of her and have a symbiotic relationship with all her creations; mineral, plant and animal. We are waking up. This is the time of the *Great Remembering.* We are tribal. We are connected. We are one.

We are linked in the beat, in the rhythm, in the sound, in the spiral, in the movement. Our natural state is to *be* Earth *grounded,* singing and dancing, in JOY.

This natural, tribal life does not exclude science or technology. In both movies there are sophisticated machines. The machines, like the body, are *forms.*

Master the *forms*, use them with *Viveka*; right discrimination, then release them to become *formless,* to *The Edge and Beyond.*

Ecology

Ecology (81) is the science that studies the interactions and interdependencies of living systems. It examines individual organism effects on self and other organisms within a system. It also looks at whole systems, acting on themselves and their interactions with other systems. When a system loses equilibrium, dramatic and profound shifts in specific organism populations occur to re-establish a new balance point.

In 1935 the *Fortymile caribou herd* was one of the largest in the world, migrating between Alaska and Canada, with a population approximating one million. By 1973 this herd was down to 6,000. This was primarily due to overharvesting by humans made easy by numerous new roads cutting across their migration paths. Other factors included predation by wolves and severe weather conditions.

In 1973 emergency measures were implemented to ban caribou hunting in an attempt to save this herd from eminent extinction. By 1990 no more than 2% of the caribou population was allowed to be harvested annually by hunters. In 1997 a wolf fertility control program was initiated and within five years the *Fortymile herd* was near 44,000.

When we have had a long enough time interval to watch and evaluate either man made manipulated interventions or natural, animal, insect or plant changes, we repeatedly see new equilibrium points develop.

As this *process* is happening, we may believe or mis-interpret the data along the way to assume or project misleading outcomes.

In the case of the caribou an inordinate amount of at-tention and intervention to decrease wolf populations has overshadowed other significant factors influenc-ing caribou population, primarily hunting. Ecology is a complex system with many variables. Our ability to accurately and correctly utilize this tool, while improv-ing, is still fraught with many difficulties and potential inaccuracies.

World Population

Currently, our planet has a human population of ap-proximately 7.06 billion. In 1350 the population was approximately 370 million. By 1804 we reached one billion, two billion by 1927, three billion by1960, four bil-lion by 1974, five billion by 1987 and six billion by 1999.

What are the consequences of this expanding popula-tion growth for the future of our species and planet? We are capable of extrapolating an outcome based on these numbers. We observe trends, crunch numbers and play with probability and statistics. Theorists sug-gest that by 2050 the population could be between, 7.5 to 10.5 billion. By 2100 they project up to as much as 16 billion or a reduction to around 6 billion. These num-bers represent projections of possibilities based on nu-merous factors.

While developed countries are experiencing either little or protracted growth, 97% of all population growth is happening in developing countries, in particular, Africa.

Is it possible or inevitable that human population is due for a natural correction or reduction similar to wild caribou herds? If so, nature would play a significant role in this correction. Certain religions may frame such a rapid population reduction as proof of Armageddon.

Quoting from the introduction of the book; *there are no accidents and no coincidences. This statement is not intended to support a deterministic view of our lives or existence. Instead it is to acknowledge our capacity to perceive patterns and then use free will to enter into a cause and or effect relationship with the pattern. When we are cause, we control our destiny. When we are effect destiny controls us.*

The only judgment that has any actual effect on us, is self-judgment. Can a religion, spiritual path or teacher, enhance our lives and our capacity to function in balance and harmony and increase our spiritual growth?

Certainly they can as long as we don't become fixated or dogmatic in our view of their value, or limit our interpretation of their intent or teaching. It is often this narrow interpretation of seeming truth that incites conflict, whether personal or between nations, and is a primary source of wars.

2012: Just Another Cycle

A cartoon shows an artisan engraving the *Mayan Calendar* (82) as he is finishing the last figure. Someone else is in the cartoon watching. The caption under the cartoon reads; *Wow, that's really going to mess with people's heads.*

In the present, we have a clear understanding of what a calendar is and how to interpret it. A calendar represents an interval of linear time. It is understood that this interval of linear time is not the beginning and end of all things, but rather a segment of varying length. That length may represent a small or large block of time.

This determination is made in reference to a time standard. Our current time standards are extrapolations that have come to us from *Newtonian*, *General Relativity* and *Quantum Physics*.

Since at present these aspects of physics have not been reconciled into a single *Unified Field Theory,* our current time standard reference points are suspect as inaccurate or questionable.

Given the sophistication of modern science to generate current time reference points, it seems curious that modern people want to imbue some presumed definitive meaning and power to an ancient calendar.

Did the ancients have some level of knowledge or technology that superseded our current abilities? This is an interesting question. At a deeper intuitive level, is there some truth to this feeling or perception about older civilizations?

We have a profound awareness of cycles, such as the number of seconds in a minute, the number of hours in a day, the number of days in a month, the number of months in a year, the number of years in a decade, century or millennium.

There are short and long cycles, as exemplified by the gestation period of animals or planetary seasons, the time it takes for Saturn to circle the Sun or the time interval between the shifting of the North and South Poles on planet Earth.

The last time the magnetic poles switched was approximately 780,000 years ago. The interval between these switches is extremely variable, ranging from forty million years at the longest, to several hundred years at the shortest.

Current evidence reflects that we are in one of these polarity shifts right now. Is the *Mayan Calendar* accurately identifying the timing for this specific current shift as it comes to completion? Popular supposition that the end of the *Mayan Calendar* is approximating the time table predicting biblical Armageddon, or the destruction of Earth is a fear based self-fulfilling projection. The *Mayan Calendar* dating is not about, *The End*; it is about one cycle ending and another cycle beginning. Some cycles have more significance or influence on our lives and *well-being* than other cycles.

The current cycle shift, reflected by the *Mayan Calendar* is a harbinger of a profound paradigm shift for the planet and all her children; human, animal, insect, vegetable and mineral.

LGBT; Lesbian, Gay, Bi-Sexual and Trans-gender (83)

Why do some people feel they are a female trapped in a male body or a male trapped in a female body?

Why is this feeling so strong that some pursue and endure the *process* of a surgical sex change? Do you have family, friends or co-workers struggling with these issues?

Our core essence, *being, soul* is neither male nor female. In our capacity as co-creators with the divine, on the journey of awakening, we generally alternate between male and female body *forms*.

This alternating gender pattern only happens within dimensions having polarity made manifest. Polarity is expressed as mixed pairs of opposites; up-down, hot-cold, man-woman, light-dark, life and death. This allows us to have a wider range of life experience to help us learn and improve our capacity for love, compassion and tolerance for ourselves and others. In our essence, we fundamentally understand that authentic love is love. This love *transcends* all limits, including any humanly *be-mi* derived restrictions.

The *form* of sexual expression, like everything, is merely a *form*. The only issue of significance is whether we as an individual, in our self-expression, place a judgment or negatively charged emotion on the *form*.

If love, associated with any act, is authentically *unconditional* than that act or *form* has neither sin nor karma attached. We are *Cause*.

The contention that the highest function and purpose of sex is reproduction is derived from *be-mi;* body, ego, mind and identity. For many, sex and orgasm is the closest experience they will ever have of a conscious connection of divine ecstatic presence.

Tantra (84) is a system of meditation and ritual. One of its aspects is the specific application of sex as a spiritual discipline. This discipline is to activate spirit as *Chi* from the root *chakra* to the crown *chakra* to induce enlightenment. Sexual intercourse actively engages the *in-flow* and *out-flow* characteristics of *Chi* as well as the *form* of the *mobius.*

In *tantric* sex physical orgasm for males is eschewed in deference to a higher manifestation of ecstatic divine connection. The premise or assertion that there is some external, arbitrary moral or ethical code defining correct sexual expression is a human mental construct, not a divine directive.

The current energy flux, induction pattern, manifesting on Earth as the magnetic poles are transposing, is a major factor influencing sexual orientation. The positive energy charge is becoming negative, *Yang* is becoming *Yin,* male is becoming female and female is becoming male. This is a natural *process*, not an imbalance or aberration but rather a refining of energy equilibrium to a new set point.

As we approach this new set point, the frequency of the magnetic shift is increasing, while the amplitude is decreasing. This is a part of the expansion and contraction *process* that defines, creates and manifests all things. It is mirrored from the microcosm to the macrocosm.

A normal consequence of this shift is increased expression of lesbian, gay, bi-sexual and trans-gender activity and interaction. Rather than being aberrant, this is actually a normal and natural progression of expanding consciousness.

Broader patterns of sexual expression are reflections, in the physical universe, of the concurrent patterns of planetary magnetic flux. This flux culminates as the switch in Earth's magnetic polarity re-establishes the female, matriarchal, Earth mother dominant energy system again. Switching of the magnetic poles is a physical dimension manifestation and reflection of the natural *process* of movement in and out of equilibrium states. From positive to negative and from male dominant to female dominant. The cycle repeats over and over.

This shifting in and out of equilibrium states is one of the fundamental parameters that affects and influences all of us.

This shifting or alternating pattern is encoded in our genes. Genes, although significant, are only one factor influencing an organism's *form* and function. *Fascia* as the connective tissue membrane surrounding all parts of the body as one continuous multi layered sac, has an influence on *form* and function that is *transcendent.*

Genes control us as *effect*. This control may seem as if it is bordering on almost absolute. This level of power and control is inherent in organic living organism systems. This control will dominate repeatedly with high precision. This dominance is proportional to our identification and actualization of self as *effect.*

For us to take back control as *cause,* we have to engage *free will* to re-activate normal function of the *fascial* membrane. When *fascia* is controlled, all *form* and function is controlled.

A tool and pathway to accomplish this is the use of *RST* and all its affiliate counterparts such as, *RMM* and *Resonant Movement Yoga* or *RMY.*

This *form* of yoga uses movement with vocal sound while interfacing the physical body with any objects in the immediate physical location. This can be done inside, but when possible I recommend *being* outside and *grounded.* The angles and stretches are generated spontaneously. A fun variation is to turn every surface into a musical instrument, primarily as a drum.

Be observant and notice the emergent planetwide *pattern* of activities and demonstrations of sound to help us *remember* and *awaken* our birthright and heritage into the *audible life stream* of spirit *Chi* as *machaneers,* (97) of *causation mechanics.* A *you tube* posting: Baikal ice live sound, playing ice like a musical instrument on a frozen lake bed and recognition of *Stonehenge being* made of ringing rocks or *blue* stones: www.dailymail.co.uk/.../why-stonehenge-prehistoric-center-rock-music are examples of this re-emergent use and understanding of sound.

Nature vs Nurture and *Epigenetics*

The differentiation of the influence of genes versus *free will* activation of *fascia,* is the age old question of the relative influence of *nature* versus *nurture.*

This has always been a difficult debate due to our fundamental lack of a reliable yard-stick or reference point to make determinations of the relative influence of *nature* versus *nurture* on us individually or as a human collective.

Nature refers to genetic determinism as the primary cause of the development of individual differences in physical and behavioral traits. Nurture identifies personal experience and social factors as dominant.

Current consensus suggests that both the genetic code of an individual and environmental factors influence development interactively.

Recent medical studies have confirmed the power of *nature,* expressed as gene influence, by studying twins or triplets separated at birth. Their findings are startling. Even when separated at birth, a high percentage of these siblings have the same health and medical problems regardless of diet and lifestyle.

They often like the same colors, foods and music. They may also be of the same religious or political affiliations.

This is powerful evidence that genes may have a much greater influence than we ever imagined. What hope, under this onslaught of such a powerful mediator of *form* and function, can we ever prevail to control much of anything?

Epigenetics involves the study of changes in the regulation of gene activity and expression that are not dependent on gene sequence. This discipline helps bring into focus the influence of environment and consciousness on gene expression.

How much does authentic *free will* influence gene expression or *causation mechanics?* The simple *free will* act of believing, wanting or visualizing an object or desired outcome is usually not sufficient to induce or create the object or specific outcome. We generally experience the truth and reality of this fact early in our lives.

Free will acts, making basic daily decisions like deciding to sleep in, play hooky from school or work, turn right or left while driving, or what clothes to wear, are examples of a pseudo, superficial aspect of *free will* that can easily delude and lull humans into a false sense of empowerment and security.

This sophisticated and complex delusion often derails people life time, after life time, from realizing they are operating as *effect* rather than *cause.*

Faith is a key to open a doorway and pass through into other dimensions. Using *free will,* to choose to *be unconditional* and not react to any stimulus with negative emotion or mental judgment, is a crucial component of *causation mechanics.* This connects our perception into awareness of the *fascial* membrane. As we increase and refine our awareness of *fascia,* we discover our inherent and natural ability to control it.

This control is not a function of the *mind-brain* activation of self-will. Self-will and *free-will* may or may not be synonymous. When they are synonymous, we are *cause,* when they are not, we are *effect.* Control comes as a function of the ability to let go and let *fascia* unwind allowing unrestricted *Chi* flow through all meridians and *chakras.* This brings true control, which is the ability to link into and be guided by the divine. This control of *fascia* allows us to *be cause.*

As *cause,* we control our destiny. In linking faith and *free will,* we increase the frequency and consistency of the ability to cross the barrier or membrane, blocking our natural ability to separate our core essence consciousness from the physical body shell into other dimensions.

Whether physically embodied, in this dimension or non-physical from other dimensions, our application of authentic faith and *free will,* catalyzes consistent experiences and awareness that firmly links us into the upward and inward spiral of expanding consciousness. This is the barometer we learn to utilize to identify whether we are functioning as *cause* rather than effect.

Earth Changes

What is the transposition of the Earth's magnetic poles influence on current planetary *Earth changes? Earth changes* (85) are changing patterns of weather including earthquakes, tornados, hurricanes, floods and other naturally occurring eco-system changes.

As the frequency of planetary focal magnetic flux is increasing, more of the planet's surface exhibits magnetic anomalies. This increase in frequency induces an increased number of *Earth changes.* At the same time that the frequency and distribution of magnetic flux is increasing, the amplitude or strength of this flux is diminishing. This diminishment is due to a more even and uniform re-distribution of Earth magnetism as we approach the end or termination of the magnetic pole shift. As the magnetic amplitude is decreasing the relative intensity of *Earth changes* become less severe.

Our ability to frame and perceive these changes as less severe is often difficult due to the extremely brief time interval of human life, as well as our recent emergence as a species on this planet, relative to geophysical history. If the Earth is approximately 4.54 billion years old than humans have emerged in the most recent last minute of this history.

Another factor that complicates or colors our perception of the importance and significance of current *Earth changes,* is the massive increase in human population from approximately 300 million in the 1300 hundreds to over 7 billion currently. Since this human population increase is widely disseminated around the world, the probability of harm to people and property increases, relative to the increasing frequency of Earth changes. The human proclivity to interpret this as meaning that *things* are getting worse, is a self-induced projection of ongoing and future events.

The increase in frequency and decrease in amplitude of *Earth changes* being induced as a natural consequence of the transposition of Earth's magnetic poles, does not suggest that we are on the cusp of a critical or devastating single catastrophic Earth event. It does suggest that we are very close to a stabilization point and that as the magnetic poles completely switch the current increase in frequency of Earth changes will dissipate to almost nothing. At the same time the amplitude or intensity of Earth changes that has already been decreasing, will also dissipate to almost nothing.

To visualize this graphically, imagine a coin that we spin on a table top. As the coin loses momentum, it starts to wobble. At first this wobble is large, its amplitude is high. At the same time its frequency is low because the wobble is slow. As the coin continues to lose momentum, we observe it quickly loosing amplitude, expressed as the strength or height of the wobble above the table's surface. As the amplitude is decreasing the coin is wobbling closer and closer to the table top. Simultaneously, we observe the speed or frequency of the wobble increasing.

Just before the coin settles motionless onto the table top, with almost no amplitude or height, the speed of its wobble is approaching its maximum frequency or velocity. A virtual instant after the coin has its lowest amplitude and highest frequency it stops completely.

Due to the significant increase in the frequency of *Earth changes,* as the current cycle is ending, combined with current Earth population, the likelihood of significant loss of property, infrastructure and life is probable. This may or may not be an ecological imperative. If a settling or balancing of human population occurs, what might we conjecture will happen to the remaining population? Any number of possibilities might be considered with varying degrees of either contracted or expanded populations. If the remaining population is too dependent on current non-sustainable technologies or natural resources that may no longer be available, their continuing survival may be in jeopardy.

At varying points within any cycle, a continuous modulation or change happens in the base, fundamental or foundational frequency of the entire system. The current reemerging foundational frequency is more resonant, harmonic and in closer alignment with our core-essence *being* as *soul*.

As this alignment develops and energetic equilibrium is in more balance, we will see a greater emergence of bi-sexuality as the new dominant, mainstream, sexual expression *form.*

Soul is *transcendent.* It is genderless. The true home of *soul* is in non-polarized dimensional space, outside the boundaries of *STEM; space-time,* energy and matter. *Soul* manifests in *space-time* with a body, to grow and learn and ultimately, to wake up and remember *what, where, how* and *why* we are here.

As *soul, here* and *now,* we are a particle of *source waking up* and consciously *reconnecting* with *fascia.* This links us into the *double-helix* of the *cause-substrate* of spirit, *Chi,* life-force, sound, *shab, logos,* voice of God, *mantra or USL.* This leads us home so we can serve life and learn to give and receive divine, *unconditional* love.

Our Earth Mother Linkage is *Being* Re-established

As the magnetic poles transpose, we are emerging into a new paradigm. This paradigm is re-emergent. Rather than actually being new, it is the manifestation of a natural cycle in transition.

The cycle is once again bringing our focus into a matriarchal; female energy phase. The current patriarchal; male energy phase is diminishing. As this happens, Earth mother linkage is *being* re-established. Earth is *Gaia*; a living conscious organism. She is our mother, we are her children. Those that insist, that this is not true and continue to try to dominate her, will find their world view and intent unsustainable.

The planet cannot support 7.06 billion people, all competing for the same non-renewable, limited resources. Will we develop alternative and renewable energy sources in time to support this level of population? If so, than what can we expect, as the world population continues to grow even larger?

Nature is cyclical, always expanding, contracting, expanding, contracting then expanding more. It has a breath or wave pulse, expressed as *Chi in-flow* and *out-flow*.

The indulgences of the developed Western nations must end and the intent of developing nations, to choose the same indulgences, is misguided and naive. Based on our current non-renewable energy resources, all humans cannot have and do not need automobiles, air-conditioning, lights that never turn off and a host of other technological conveniences. The instant gratification, petulant, childish mentality, being fostered in the world today, is a reflection of our egocentricity as a species.

We are *Avatar,* hiding in our disconnected, trance induced human consciousness. Our birthright and heritage, as *Avatar,* is to re-awaken our natural symbiotic, psychic connection with all Earth mothers; gems, plants, insects, animals, fellow humans, Earth spirit *beings*, as well as all corporeal, material consciousness *forms*, as well as all non-corporeal energy consciousness *forms*, throughout the universe.

Warp Drive; Faster than Light Speed Travel is not Through Worm Holes

Mankind has attempted to find proof of alien life. Scientists have speculated that life, if it exists outside Earth, must be rare. This is a projection of their own limited perception of this possibility or probability. The universe is teeming with life. Physical stars are extremely far apart. This is part *of intelligent design.*

I am not referring to the term *intelligent design* as usurped by Christian theology to replace their conceptualization of creationism. I am referring to *intelligent design* as the presence and guidance of divine intent and will.

If the universe is teeming with life, how are we to ever find it, get to it or communicate with it? The very best current science has no viable options to solve this conundrum. The probability, that we will someday reach these stars, by making physical, metal space ships, that will move through wormholes by collapsing the fabric of *space-time* is science fiction at best.

Warp drive (86) or faster than light speed travel, is and has always been attainable, as a function of awakening consciousness. It is an essential step in our remembering and awakening journey.

The universe offers us the challenge to find a way to find each other in every consciousness *form*, planet to planet, throughout the universe, dimension to dimension. It is up to us whether we step up to the plate and accept the challenge.

Kardashev Scale

In 1964 a Russian astronomer Nikolai Kardashev developed a theoretical model for categorizing a civilizations technological advancement relative to the amount of energy it is able to generate and consume. The primary scale has three levels. Currently Earth isn't even on the scale as it has a designation of type 0. A type 0 civilization is still dependent on the consumption of organic matter for energy like, wood, coal, oil and gas. A type I civilization is able to harness all the power of a single planet, approximately 10 billion megawatts; 4×10^{12} watts. A type II civilization can harness the energy of a sun or approximately 100 billion, billion megawatts; 4×10^{26} watts. A type III civilization can harness the energy of an entire galaxy; 4×10^{37} watts.

The Large Hadron Collider or LHC requires about 120 MW or megawatts to operate. A megawatt is one million watts. This is the power required to drive two particle beams close to the speed of light in opposing directions. The resulting collisions have been characterized as *mini big bangs.*

Scientists have speculated that these collisions may induce microscopic black holes or worm holes. If present, they would be extremely unstable with a very fast decay rate.

If it takes 120 MW of energy for a super collider to make an unstable microscopic worm hole, how much energy might it take to make an actual stable worm hole for interstellar travel? Scientists conjecture, if a stable worm hole could ever actually be sustained, it would require a level III civilization, able to harness the power of an entire galaxy. This makes worm holes an unlikely viable option for meaningful interstellar space travel.

In the Kardashev scale the only variable used for evaluating a civilization is its technology relative to energy consumption. Scientists have acknowledged that our theoretical projections of the defining characteristics of more advanced civilizations may be completely wrong. Carl Sagan suggested an expansion of the scale to include the amount of information, quantified in bits, available to a civilization. This expansion adds mental capacity to the scale. Using the alphabet as symbols to differentiate the amounts of bits available; A represents 10^6 bits. He identified 1973 Earth as having 10^{13} bits of information available and a Z level civilization as having 10^{31} bits available.

This addition to the Kardashev scale by Sagan is as much a speculative abstraction about advanced civilizations as the original scale itself. As such it may also be right on the mark, or not even close.

Another criteria to reflect about civilization, which is inherent from a spiritual perspective, is *the ability of any given life form to live in harmony with itself, its own species and all other life forms.*

I preferentially use this definition and contend that it is a more authentic parameter for framing advancement of any given civilization. This criteria may or may not have any technology or energy consumption associated with it.

Another expansion of the scale includes type IV civilizations, harnessing the energy of the entire universe; 10^{45} watts and type V civilizations able to use the *multiverse* or other higher order dimensions of existence.

If there is technology or energy consumption at these levels, I agree with Zoltan Galantai who contends that such civilizations would be undetectable, as their functional abilities would be indistinguishable from nature. They would be true masters of *causation mechanics.*

The premise that their use of energy is dependent on the mundane conceptualization of energy as reflected by watts or technology as reflected by machines is a misnomer. They are functionally able to utilize the spirit life force *Chi* emanating from the *un-manifest no-thing* dimensions.

As humans choose to live in harmony with themselves, their own species, and all other life forms, they become able to actualize personal and collective spiritual awakening through utilization of tools like *RST* and *RMM.* There is no past, there is no future, we all live in the eternal now.

Faster than light speed intergalactic, inter-dimensional travel is a function of awakening consciousness. It is our birth right as *soul*.

Where are these advanced civilizations? Let me share a little secret. They are *here, now*. Some exist in the dimensions of *STEM; space-time,* energy and matter. Most exist in other dimensions.

We are them and they are us. The difference is that some of them-us are awakened, while others are still awakening; on the verge of remembering, to take our place as collective *soul*. Humans on planet Earth are primarily in the latter group.

The Road to El Dorado

A Disney cartoon movie titled; *The Road to El Dorado* (87)*,* is about the Spaniards coming to the *New World* in search of new discoveries, fame and fortune. In the opening credits, there is a scene where Earth is seen as a globe from a distance. As the camera pans in, it shows pyramids all over the planet with beams of light projecting out of their tops.

The beams coalesce from all the pyramids to *form* a grid or matrix of light surrounding the planet's surface. This matrix of light is a beacon that projects both into the furthest reaches of the physical universe, as well as all non-physical, multi-dimensional spaces. The light functions as both a communication and transport device. The critical component for this *light grid matrix* to be activated is the utilization of the correct *resonant* frequencies of sound.

This beacon establishes the signal that, *we are here,* and that, we are ready, once again, to re-establish the connection with these inner and outer worlds and dimensions.

Pictures both from space and on Earth demonstrate that this planet is actually covered with real physical pyramids widely dispersed across its surface. They have been identified in Indonesia, Australia, Bosnia, throughout China, and India. Many of these are much larger and older than the uncovered pyramids in Egypt, Mexico, Central and South America. The majority of them are unlikely to ever be excavated due to their age and depth underneath mountains of soil and rock.

With the development of the telegraph, human capability for transmission and reception of an intelligent signal, both immediately and everywhere on the planet, went from zero to one-hundred percent, in *the blink of an eye.*

This virtual miracle was hailed by all people, and *overnight,* the telegraph was accepted and integrated into the world. This was accepted and integrated so rapidly that people didn't take the opportunity or really didn't seem to have the time, to reflect and contemplate on the amazing ramifications of the discovery and implementation of a *planetary telegraphic grid.*

In The Blink of an Eye

A brief review of communication technology takes us sequentially from the telegraph, to the telephone, to the beginnings of many *forms* of wireless applications.

As we observe the principle in action; *from the contracted, to the expanded, to the more expanded,* after the telephone came radio, television, computers, cell phones and *the world-wide internet web.* All of this technology is dependent on physical machines.

The planetary *light-grid matrix,* although augmentable with machine technology, is not dependent on it. This significant difference introduces the concept of *spiritual technology.* What is the fundamental difference between *spiritual technology* and regular technology? Both *forms* of technology are part of the same continuum, but for *spiritual technology* there is the elimination of the necessity of a physical machine interface.

Physical pyramids that were deemed critically necessary, and used historically to create, and functionally activate the planet's *light-grid matrix* are no longer essential. To light and maintain the Earth's *light-grid matrix* does not require any physical machine. It can be turned on and maintained as a function of either individual or group consciousness.

As we approach and maintain the *critical mass* energy of expanded consciousness necessary for the re-establishment of the *matrix,* what it is and what it offers us becomes more and more accessible to everyone.

Throughout time, individuals have mastered faster than light speed travel. It has always been a function of expanded personal consciousness and not the result of any machine technology. Historically, this has always been the domain of a small, select group of *Hu*-mans.

Spirit as resonant, harmonic sound establishes the re-induction of the planetary *light-grid matrix*. A frequency is established, that potentiates the signal, for faster than light speed, communication and transport.

The presence of the planetary *light-grid matrix* makes it easier for anyone to utilize faster than light speed applications.

With modest discipline, for those who choose to engage the *process* of expanding consciousness, these faster than light speed applications, may no longer be the exclusive domain of the few, but now the many.

Comparing the current, increased ease of information availability and dissemination, with access to the *worldwide internet web,* as compared to before the webs existence, is a good reflection of the influence and potential of the planetary *light-grid matrix*, before and after its activation.

The Prime Directive

In the science fiction, TV and movie series *Star Trek,* there is a guiding principle that must be adhered to by all members of the *Federation of Planets.* This principle is called, *The Prime Directive.* It states that no advanced civilization, on encountering any newly discovered inhabited planet or sentient life *form* is to have any communication or contact.

The contact is only restricted if the newly discovered life *form* does not have a planetary knowledge of and a functional *Warp Drive;* faster than light speed transport system.

The rationale for this directive is to not interfere with the natural growth and development of any awakening civilization.

The full activatation of the planetary light grid in 2012, although possible, was not achieved. We are continuing to increase its field strength. The inevitability of the *critical mass* tipping point for full activation is close at hand. The image of the pyramids from the movie, *The Road to El Dorado,* visually represents actual historic facts.

The ancients that built pyramids, all over our planet, knew, understood and utilized them to activate the planetary *light-grid matrix* and engage faster than light speed communication and transport.

The *Mayan Calendar* identifies the end of one planetary cycle and the beginning of another, linked to the transposition of the Earth's magnetic poles. It also predicts the potential initiation point in linear time for re-establishment of the planetary *light-grid matrix.*

The grid is a harbinger, not of new knowledge and discovery but of the *Great Remembering* and *Awakening.* The cycle is renewed once again, from the *contracted; less than*, knowledge and awareness base, to the *expanded; more than*, knowledge and awareness base. This is the wave or pulse quality of life and consciousness in action, as *in-flow* and *out-flow.*

Burning Man and *Earth Dance* to Re-ignite the Planetary *Light-Grid Matrix*

Burning Man (88) is an annual event, in the NW corner of Nevada, held every August. Over fifty-thousand people from all over the planet come together for one week. They create an intentional community with no single focus, although fine *arts,* in their many and varied *forms* are evident everywhere. The one dominant creative expression is music and dance.

The majority of this music, played from dawn to dusk, on numerous stages, is in the genre of *Electronic-Techno-Trance* or *EDM;* electronic dance music.

Burning Man has ten guiding principles: *radical inclusion, gifting, decommodification;* which is creating a social environment in which commodities are neither sold nor advertised, *radical self-reliance, radical self-expression, communal effort, civic responsibility, leaving no trace, participation and immediacy.*

Over the years, I have been observing an interesting phenomenon triggered by *Burning Man* and potentiated by *Earth Dance* (89) which occurs approximately one month after *Burning Man* every year.

Earth Dance is the largest yearly global synchronized music and dance celebratory expression. It has up to five hundred simultaneous events occurring in over eighty countries and is growing. *Earth Dance,* like *Burning Man,* has a predominance of *Electronic-Techno-Trance* music or *EDM* (90) at its foundation.

It is neither accidental nor coincidental that this *Electronic* music is so prevalent. This type of music, in an ever expanding array of creative cross-linked sub-genres has been experiencing a global renaissance of popularity and acceptance, in particular with younger generations. A good portion of this music has very powerful conscious and subconscious cues that link the listener to expanded states of consciousness and awareness.

Much of this electronic music has and is being seeded on this planet from other parts of the universe and other dimensions. It has been catalytic in drawing younger generations into a re-awakening-initiation of our *Earth grounded* and *Tribal* nature, heritage and birthright.

Join Us, Grounded to the Earth, Singing and Dancing

To be *grounded* to the Earth means to have actual physical contact between the body and the spirit-*Chi* energy field of planet Earth as Gaia, our living conscious mother. The full range of Earth *Chi* is much wider than electricity, and has energy gradients that expand beyond the currently known or understood electro-magnetic spectrum.

We are *grounded* when barefoot or barefoot wearing a leather moccasin with the Earth or an Earth *grounded* material on the outside. Any natural material, foot covering, from cotton, to wool, to wood or other plant fibers, like woven grass are *grounded.*

Most modern footwear with rubber or plastic soles, act as an almost perfect insulator, separating the wearer, from Earth *Chi*. Dirt, sand, rock, brick or grass outside is *grounded*. Natural material; tile, slate, brick, marble, wood or 100% wool carpet or rugs are also *grounded*. Uncovered cement slabs decrease Earth *Chi*. Synthetic carpets reduce *Chi* access substantially.

Participants of *Burning Man, Earth Dance* or any other event with dancing and music, as well as any spiritual gatherings, should be mindful and observant, specifically in relation to the ability to feel and experience the natural *in-flow* and *out-flow* of *Chi* through the body.

This is the feeling or transmission of *Chi*-spirit-energy through the Earth, into the body, into the inner world dimensions and then out of the inner world dimensions, out through the body, back into the Earth.

At *Burning Man 2012*, many of the music stages had synthetic carpet on the ground to reduce duct. Participants were often dancing with boots or tennis shoes with rubber soles. This does not stop us from enjoying ourselves and feeling some of the morphic field energy generated by a group of dancing people. It does, however, significantly reduce our ability as a group to transmit an energy signal through the Earth which is a primary function of events like *Burning Man*.

At *Burning Man*, there is a spark or signal generated, of varying energy magnitude that lights a fuse. The magnitude of this signal is in direct proportion to how many participants are *grounded*.

One month after *Burning Man* is *Earth Dance*. As the lit fuse from *Burning Man* connects to *Earth Dance* events all over the world, combined with the charge of *Chi* energy generated from *Earth Dance* itself, ignition is induced. This ignition is the *Critical Mass* needed to re-ignite the planetary *light-grid matrix*.

Over the last several years prior to 2012 we had successfully been blinking the planetary matrix. In 2012 we had the potential to ignite it and keep it turned on. This potential was not actualized due to the use of synthetic carpets and a majority of participants wearing rubber soled shoes effectively blocking the critical *grounding* necessary for full *light-grid matrix* induction.

We do not need physical pyramids or any other physical machine or object to re-ignite the planetary *light-grid matrix*. All we need is *Chi*-consciousness generated by *Hu*-mans, *grounded to the Earth, Singing and Dancing.* Share this message with your family, friends and co-workers. *Critical Mass, the Hundredth Monkey* effect is ready for full activation and ignition. This is a function of personal and group *free will* action.

Dr. Seuss; *Horton Hears a Who*

Dr. Seuss, (91) one of the great spiritual teachers of our times, wrote many children's stories with embedded spiritual truths or lessons. Much of Theodor Seuss Geisel's children's stories were construed to mask social and political commentary. Dr. Seuss never admitted this, but did acknowledge that there were moral lessons in his works, not so much intentionally, but co-incidental to his writings. Would he, if asked, acknowledge a conscious intent and awareness of deeper spiritual musings to be gleaned from his stories?

Numerous books, stories, TV shows, movies and music are filling in details, of what is *really going on*, linking pieces and transmitting this information to all of us either overtly or covertly. The writers or producers of this information have varying degrees of conscious or unconscious awareness, as to the true-deeper meaning suggested by their works.

In the story, *Horton Hears a Who*, (92) Dr. Seuss transmits an amazing spiritual insight, whether consciously or from the deepest recesses of his inner core, *soul being*. Dr. Seuss at some level realized that vocal sound was an integral and essential part of establishing our conscious link with both the distant stars and inner divine worlds.

He offers the suggestion, reflected in the specific children's story, *Horton Hears a Who,* that we can magnify or activate our voice, to make this profound connection. In the story, one of his characters uses a large funnel or cone to magnify his voice as he shouts; *we are here, we are here*. Through this *conical spiral*, the sound is potentiated.

The *conical spiral* is one half of the *double helix,* which is the *form* used by *source* to transmit its essence spirit as sound across the membrane dividing the *un-manifest* realm into polarized manifest dimensions.

The critical importance of the use of a cone by the *Who* from *Whosville* to make it possible for the elephant Horton to hear him, is a reflection of the critical function of the *conical spiral*, as half of the *double helix* to transmit spirit as sound in a clockwise spiral *out-flow* into manifest dimensions.

It is the other half of the *double helix*, transmitting spir-it as sound in a counter-clockwise spiral *in-flow* that awakening *soul* must link into and ride back across the membrane dividing manifest dimensions into the *un-manifest, no-thing* realm, home of *source.*

The cone is the medium necessary for Horton the el-ephant to hear the *Who.* Horton relays the message to everyone that there really are people living, on the speck of dust, on the clover flower he is holding. No one believes the elephant, nor is willing to be patient enough to pause and get close enough, to listen care-fully enough, to confirm that the elephant is telling the truth.

This is happening in the modern world. Many people are neither willing nor interested enough, to prove or demonstrate for themselves, what *is, really going on.* Dr. Seuss's use of the title, *Horton Hears a Who,* is of particular importance and has a powerful subcon-scious effect on the reader. The word *Who* is almost identical to a syllable, that comes to us from sacred, *USL;* universal sound language.

Sacred, *USL;* Universal Sound Language

We all know and speak this language. It is not lost, but merely forgotten or suppressed. We may believe that it neither exists, nor is it actually accessible to us as in-dividuals. This is a self-projected illusion of disconnect and is easily overcome and disproven with personal utilization of syllables of the sacred ancient sound lan-guage.

Syllables we still remember, that are universal, regardless of our specific spoken language, manifest as crying, laughing, sighing, wails, moans, many other natural guttural sounds or clicks, as well as all the sounds made during sex.

This language is manifest as *mantra*. *Mantra* is the specific use of a vocal sound that creates a resonant harmonic with our physical body that induces vibration, unwinding body *fascia*. This causes a state of energetic equilibrium. This equilibrium state potentiates healing of the physical, emotional, mental and spiritual *being*. It is also a tool for expanding consciousness, enlightenment and faster than light speed travel. The word *Who* from Dr. Seuss is a very close approximation of the *mantra HU.*

Like the more commonly known *mantra AUM,* that many people in the West have been exposed to through Eastern mystical, spiritual teachings, both of these *mantras* are part of *USI* As *Hu-*mans it is our birthright to remember this sacred language and be able, once again, to fully integrate and use it.

Although we can use this language to potentiate or manifest personal self-serving desires, this application is self-limiting. It is self-limiting because used in this way, we induce a *cause* and effect feedback loop. This is *Newton's Second Law of Mechanics or Motion;* for every action there is an equal and opposite reaction. Our *transcendent* heritage is to use the sacred sound language as a vehicle or conduit of divine rather than personal will.

AUM or OM

AUM (93) is part of the sound language at a frequency, vibrational rate emanating from within the *space-time* continuum. It is part of the manifest universe. *Being* manifest, *Aum* is a *form.* By definition it is limited.

HU

HU (94) is part of the sound language at a frequency, vibrational rate emanating from outside the *space-time* continuum. It is part of the *un-manifest* universe, coming from the furthest reaches of the *no-thing* realm. *Being un-manifest, Hu* is not a *form.* It is *formless* and unlimited. It crosses the final membrane, edge of the *space-time* continuum to establish a two way connection link between manifest and *un-manifest* dimensions. Looking at *Hu*-man history, the *HU* is found in all religious and spiritual teachings.

Examples come from the *Druids,* ancient *Buddhism, Indigenous-Native* cultures, *Shamanism* and early *Christianity.*

The *Mayan Tree of Life* is a symbolic depiction of creation. In the center is planet Earth or the physical dimension, above it are 13 levels and below it are 9 levels. The supreme deity or creator, the *source* from which all consciousness springs is *Hu nab ku.* It is neither surprising nor coincidental that the ancient Mayans understood and utilized *HU.*

In modern times, an ancient teaching called *ECKAN-KAR; the religion of light and sound,* has made a valiant effort to introduce *HU* back into the public domain. *ECKANKAR* (95) deserves a standing ovation for this herculean effort.

It is important to understand, *HU* belongs to no one person, entity, religion or organization. *HU* is not property or proprietary. *ECKANKAR* neither claims ownership, nor creation of *HU.*

ECKANKAR recognizes *HU's* value and importance as a vehicle for expanded consciousness and continues to authentically offer it freely to the world and all its inhabitants. *HU* transcends all religions and spiritual teachings.

At the beginning of an *RST* therapy session, I have my patient start by *toning HU.* I then link my voice to the patient's voice *toning HU,* as a resonant-harmonic.This immediately allows access and utilization of the full depth, richness and complexity, yet simplicity of *USL.* This is a *process* of stepping out of the way, to function as a conduit allowing *Chi,* as spirit sound to do what it will. I bring no intent, nor project any specific outcome on my patient.

With the ability to see and feel *Chi* spirit sound, I verbally share its visual characteristics. This reinforces what already *is,* without an attempt to control or direct anything. This accelerates unwinding of the physical body fascial membrane. This induces energetic equilibrium, balance and healing of mind-body and spirit.

Since *HU* exists in frequency bands that are part of all dimensions both manifest and *un-manifest*, it also offers an exceptional tool for expanding consciousness and engaging faster than light speed travel.

We are not the body; the body is only a shell. Our true essence, spirit, consciousness, unit of awareness, is *Soul. Soul* travels faster than light and crosses through the last manifest membrane into *un-manifest*, non-physical dimensions. There is a direct relationship between the unwinding of physical *fascia,* its permeability, the free flow of *Chi*-spirit sound reflected as light, and our ability to travel faster than light.

The Form is not The Way, The Way is The Way. The Form can lead or point to The Way, so master it, than release it and remember The Form is not The Way, The Way is The Way.

I do not endorse or advocate any specific *form*, system, religion, philosophy or theory. I do advocate that anyone use *any form* that helps them move from a more contracted perception and awareness linkage on the downward spiral, to a more expanded perception moving up the spiral. Be cautious how much power or authority you give or imbue to any *form*.

All *forms* are intended to be mastered and released, to be used to derive the greatest and highest benefit available through divine rather than self-will. *Forms* are used as stepping stones to cross the last barrier membrane edge of the *space-time* dimension into the *formless beyond*.

The *Proof is in the Pudding*

Sound is the cause substrate creating and controlling everything. It is the divine logos. It is the voice of God or Word and is available to all of us.

This availability comes to each and every one of us, only if we actively vocalize *mantras. Mantras* as syllables of *USL,* successfully activate the resonant, harmonic, sound, vibration and frequency that alters personal perception, awareness and consciousness into the ever wider and more expanded band-width of possible perception and reality. It is a matter of *free will,* whether or not we use it. *The proof is in the pudding.*

The use of vocal sound induces the conical shape that is the beginning of the *mobius;* the figure eight that is twisted in three dimensions, resembling an infinity symbol.

Looking at our essence as a superimposed *sphere* on the physical body, the reference to *Chi* flowing from the bottom up and the top down is now superseded by *inside-out* and *outside-in,* which encompasses all three-hundred and sixty degrees of both vertical and horizontal aspects of the *sphere.*

Visualize a *sphere.* Imagine that this *sphere* is a ball you are holding in your hands. From the surface of this ball, any line drawn into the center of the ball is from the *outside-in.* Any line drawn from the center of the ball to its surface is from the *inside-out.* Planet Earth is a *sphere,* does it have a top or bottom? The answer is no. We frame our experience on Earth with the belief that it has a top and bottom.

This is true because we orient our relationship on the planet's surface using the equator and the magnetic poles as reference points. The equator serves as the flat surface and the poles from that surface can be projected or perceived as up and down.

Looking at or examining any other celestial body in the universe, we can only identify its spherical nature and the properties of *inside-out* and *outside-in*. It is only when an equator is identified relative to magnetic polarity that reference to up and down is applicable.

Our fundamental essence as *soul*, existing outside the boundaries of *STEM*, can be equated or visualized as a *sphere*.

When this *sphere* is energetically linked to our physical body *form*, having density, it pulls the *sphere* to conform to the physicality of the body making the *sphere* egg-shaped.

As the twin spirals of the *double helix* of *Chi*, spirit, sound hit body *fascia* as *in-flow* and *out-flow* the energy egg becomes a *torus*. This shape looks like a donut, having a central hole stretched to conform to the physicality of an object, through which *Chi* flows. The research of *Stanley N. Tenen* is a brilliant expose' on the *torus*, derived from his work transcribing the Hebrew text of Genesis, as a mathematical cipher describing the *process* of creation.

The twin primary aspects or qualities of *Chi* as spirit energy are sound and light. Sound is the cause substrate. It is the essence of *source.* As *source* essence spirit sound enters *space-time* it manifests as particles or clusters of particles with varying degrees of density.

An object like a rock has high density, while air has low density. Air, as an object in *space-time,* is still a physical object.

The saying that *feelings or thoughts are things,* although considered an abstraction, is actually correct. Feelings and thoughts only exist in the manifest dimensions of *space-time.* Everything within the polarized dimensions of *space-time* have density, they are actual things.

The difference between the relative density of rock and air is as great as the difference between the relative density of air and feelings.

The difference between the relative density of feelings and thoughts represents another order of magnitude. Creation has no density, no particles and is not matter. Manifestation has density, it has particles and it is matter.

Light is the reflection of sound made manifest as sound induces matter. The vocal sounds and syllables of *USL* induce a resonant harmonic on *fascia.* This is *Chi* spirit as the dual spinning spirals. of *in-flow* spinning counterclockwise and *out-flow* spinning clockwise, hitting *fascia.* The impact of these twin spirals on *fascia* causes the spirals to twist, inducing the *form* of a *mobius.* The *mobius,* being a figure eight twisted in three dimensions, continues its twisting to become a *double helix.* The *double helix* of *Chi* spirit as sound and reflected light travels through and permeates all *fascia.* When there is no twisting of *fascia* to disrupt the flow of *Chi,* the body remains in a state of energetic equilibrium.

Chi spirit sound crosses into the physical dimension, manifesting all physical *forms* as objects. Objects having different physical densities reflect different bands or rays of the light spectrum. Only some objects can be seen with physical senses. One way to describe the fundamental difference between physical objects as *forms* is a difference of frequency or vibration.

One *form* manifests as DNA; the building block of all organic life. It is not a coincidence that this most fundamental organic *form* has the double helical shape.

DNA's primary role, as an essential and basic component of all organic living *forms*, makes it the perfect object *form* to reflect or emulate the *double helix* of *Chi* spirit.

A Mobius-(Infinity) Passes Through the Singularity of Black Holes

Aspects of *Quantum physics* and *General Relativity* have been demonstrated in the lab but their respective mathematical proofs, at the singularity of a black hole, give the answer *Infinity*. Physicists speculate that this could not be the correct answer. From their perspective, there must be a flaw in the equations, answer, or both. A different interpretation demonstrates that the answer *Infinity* is correct.

The singularity of a black hole is the point through which that emanating from the *no-thing, un-manifest* realm, crosses the threshold of the singularity to become manifest as matter.

This emanation is the *cause* substrate, spirit, living *audible life stream*, sound, *shab*, *logos* or voice of God, which exists in frequency bands stretching from the audible, to the inaudible, to the super-audible, into frequencies that can no longer be framed as frequencies, neither perceived nor understood from any linear, mind, *space-time* oriented consciousness.

The sacred sound creates and manifests the vibrating strings of *String Theory*. These strings *form* the membranes that manifest as either energy or things, in many and varied *forms* throughout *space-time*.

That which *IS* on the other side of black hole singularities is devoid of any *space-time,* energy or matter. The mind and its current modern science derivatives are manifestations of *form*. These *forms* optimized, successfully bring us to the brink or edge of *space-time*.

They bring us to the singularity of a black hole. As *forms* they cannot bring us through to the other side. The other side, *being formless*, can only be approached as we surrender and release the mind from its ever vigilant control of our consciousness, re-establishing the link and control back to essence as *soul*.

Descartes

Descartes (96) the father of modern Western philosophy, in his preeminent axiom stated; *I think, therefore I am*. This premise has been instrumental in supporting and perpetuating our mind, super-mind, brain driven understanding of self and the universe.

From the other side of the *space-time singularity* of a black hole the axiom is; *I am, therefore I think.* Consciousness and consciousness alone *transcends* the *mind-brain*, crossing the final barrier, membrane, edge of *space-time* into the infinite void of *no-thing*.

Modern astronomy is documenting that at the center of all galaxies there is a large black hole, as well as numerous smaller black holes dispersed throughout. Black holes exist at the smallest Quantum sub-atomic particle level, all the way to the macro level of the largest stars and the furthest reaches of the physical universe. This is the axiom of *as-above - so-below* and *as -within - so-without,* being reflected through all levels and layers of *space-time,* energy and matter.

The *Big Bang* was the location of the first primordial black hole in the known universe. The singularity of this black hole was the point through which all *space-time,* energy and matter were created and made manifest.

From the infinite *no-thing* realm, that overlaps all *space-time,* is *space-time* made. Physicists state that from the *Big Bang,* which started as an infinitely small point that all the energy and matter of our entire universe sprang forth in an instant. S*pace-time* appeared at the instant of the *Big Bang.* The *mind-brain* can almost get this but ultimately fails, as it flails and twists in a feeble attempt to understand. Imagine the *Big Bang* as spirit *Chi* passing through the first primordial black hole functioning as a holographic projector. As the *audible life stream* of spirit passed through its singularity it manifested all *STEM; space-time,* energy and matter.

The transition of the *un-manifest* hologram as *source* passing through this first primordial black hole holographic projector, shattered the *un-manifest* hologram into manifest holographic fragments. Each fragment *being* a miniature replica of the original hologram. The original hologram existing in the *no-thing, un-manifest* realm is *source* or God.

It is the passage of the hologram's essence as spirit sound, both entering and simultaneously manifesting *space-time,* energy and matter that fractures the original *un-manifest* hologram into the fragments of itself, now made manifest as miniature replicas. Each fragment is essence, it is *soul.* This holographic fracturing is what induces the presence of black holes throughout all levels and layers of *space-time* and is made manifest throughout all polarized dimensions.

From the infinite *no-thing* realm, that *overlaps* all *space-time,* is *space-time* made. The answer to the equations of *Quantum Physics and Relativity Theory* at the singularity of a black hole must be *infinity*. From *no-thing* comes everything.

Everything, being manifest, defines each thing as a *form*. A *form* has a border or edge. It is encapsulated in a membrane. A *form* by definition has boundaries and limits. All *forms* are finite. *Space-time,* energy and matter are the components of which all polarized dimensions manifest. They are individually and collectively *forms*. A *form* is always limited, it is less than. Although it may seem that the physical dimension is infinite, this is actually only a theoretical supposition.

As we come to understand the nature of *space-time,* energy and matter as *forms,* we know and understand that they are limited and finite.

That which is *infinite* exists on the other side of black hole singularities. On the other side there is *no-thing.* Nothing is manifest. There are no *forms.* There is no *space-time,* energy or matter. Black holes are dimensional portals.

String Theory Re-visited

String Theory mathematically extrapolates the presence of eleven dimensions. First is a point; this is one dimension. Second is a line that can move forward or backwards, as well as side to side, this is two dimensions. Third is a line that can also go up and down, or in and out; this is three dimensions. Fourth is the variable of time; this is four dimensions. These first four describe the dimensions of *space-time.*

They are *forms*; structures and systems that take us to the final or last membrane between the manifest and the *un-manifest*, to the singularity of all black holes but not through them.

String Theory mathematically extrapolates the presence of seven additional dimensions. Many *String theorists* suggest that these other dimensions are actually parallel universes with bizarre and often inexplicable properties or characteristics. What if these seven additional dimensions are not parallel universes but actually different dimensions? What if these dimensions exist on the other side of black hole singularities?

These extra non-physical dimensions would no longer conform to or have any of the qualities or properties of the manifest physical dimension.

By definition, they have neither edges nor membranes as perceived or conceived from any physical *space-time* dimensional conceptualization. Any mathematical extrapolation of their presence or properties can only bring us to edge of the last membrane dividing *STEM; space-time,* energy and matter from the *no-thing, un-manifest* dimension.

As such these mathematical figures derived from and within *STEM* can neither take us through this membrane nor give us an accurate glimpse of what is on the other side. The math will however give us confusing and bizarre data with little or no meaningful, coherent or usable information.

The seven extra dimensions of *String Theory* cannot *be* understood from a mind and time driven linear framework or physical experimental model or test.

The one concept that can be applied as an abstraction is that all dimensions, whether on the energy and physical side of a black hole or whether on the *no-thing*, non-energy, non-physical side, are differentiated as a function of sound, frequency and vibration. The catch is that other than as a mathematical abstraction, as postulated by *String Theory*, the proof or evidence of sound, frequency and vibrational states existing at all on the *un-manifest* side of black holes and being differentiated from the sound, frequency and vibration states on the manifest side of black holes, has no possible physically objective confirmable experimental test.

It does however have a subjective confirmable experimental test. This gives modern physicists pause. They suggest that *String Theory,* under these circumstances is not a scientifically sound provable theory but can only be relegated to the category of a philosophy.

Gravity is Like an Ice-berg, it is an Extra-Dimensional Force

String Theorists suggest that gravity is an extra-dimensional force. Gravity has continued to elude modern physicists in their attempts to explain the nature of reality and reconcile *Quantum Mechanics and Relativity.* Gravity is identified as one of the four fundamental forces of nature along with electromagnetism and what is referred to as the strong and weak force.

Gravity acts between all objects with physical mass in the universe, regardless of distance. Einstein elegantly suggested that gravity was induced as a function of objects having mass warping the fabric of *space-time.*

The electromagnetic forces act between all electrically charged particles. This includes electricity, magnetism and light. The strong force binds neutrons and protons together in the cores of atoms. The weak force induces what is called beta decay. This is the conversion of a neutron to a proton and an electron into an antineutrino. Additional particles called *strange* ones are also produced. These fundamental forces of nature have been unified, within the same mathematical structure, with the exception of gravity.

Imagine that gravity is like an iceberg. The portion of gravity supposedly induced by objects with mass acting on each other is the tip of this iceberg. Historically the only portion of gravity that we perceive or describe, in the physical universe, where mass exists, is this tiny portion sticking into the physical universe out of the singularity of black holes.

The majority of gravity is on the other side of black holes, in the *no-thing*, non-physical dimension, from where it exerts the majority of its influence on the physical universe. Not only does this explain why it has such a powerful effect in the physical universe but also why we can neither fully understand nor quantify it. Will evidence of the presence of elusive *gravity waves* help to reconcile current discrepancies in our understanding of *space-time*? As we are able to quantify *gravity waves* will we demonstrate that they are coming out of the singularities of black holes?

Cosmic Inflation

The observable universe is both *isotropic;* appearing similar in all directions and *homogeneous;* having the same background cosmic microwave radiation and temperature everywhere. The *Big Bang Theory* does not adequately explain these properties of the physical universe. *Inflation* is a theory that does. It postulates that immediately after the *Big Bang* the universe expanded much faster than the speed of light. For this to occur requires a *cosmologic constant*, deemed to be a large vacuum energy. *Inflation theorists* use the analogy of a rapidly inflating balloon. That which is within this balloon or on its surface, as *STEM,* is neither moving nor expanding faster than the speed of light.

Only the balloon edge or membrane is expanding faster than the speed of light. Remember, from *String Theory,* vibrating strings coalesce to form *branes* or membranes. It is the *form* of the membrane that is the template matrix for life force spirit *Chi* to fill, which then manifests as things or objects in the domain or dimension of *STEM.*

Consider the image analogy of *inflation* as an expanding balloon, literally. The balloon is a *form.* A *form* has an edge or membrane. A *form* defines a limit; it is less than. The universe, as *STEM* being manifest, is finite. That which is infinite is on the other side of black hole singularities as the *no-thing, un-manifest* dimension.

All of *STEM; space-time,* energy and matter were made manifest as the action of the *cosmologic constant* induced an increase in velocity, exponentially accelerating expansion of the physical universe. This *inflation* period lasted from 10^{-36} seconds after the *Big Bang* to sometime between 10^{-33} and 10^{-32} seconds.

After *inflation* a new equilibrium state was established and the universe has continued to expand at a much slower rate. I conjecture that the *cosmologic constant* must be derived from all gravitational influences combined as one numerical constant. Gravity, as an extra-dimensional force, emanating from the *un-manifest, no-thing* realm, into the dimension of polarity, both when the physical universe originally manifested, as well as in present time, represents the largest part of this *cosmologic numerical constant.*

The vacuum energy that is the *cosmologic constant* is the push pull, *out-flow, in-flow* wave *form* of gravity as it passes back and forth through the singularity of black holes.

Could this gravity wave *form* have attributes of both attraction and *repulsion?* Is the *repulsion* component a type of *antigravity* or something else? The attractive force induces *in-flow. In-flow* induces contraction. The repulsive force induces *out-flow. Out-flow* induces expansion. Expansion and contraction start and stop at the final membrane interface between *STEM* and dimensions that are *un-manifest.*

Chi, qi, ki, spirit, life force, *source* essence, audible life stream, the word or voice of God and *shab* or sound current are all synonyms. Physical things or objects are either carriers or conduits for spirit. This living sound energy spirit stream creates, manifests and sustains everything. It is the *out-flow, clockwise* spiral wave *form* coming from and through all overlapping *un-manifest* inner dimensions into *STEM.* Simultaneously it is the *in-flow, counter-clockwise* spiral wave *form* coming from and through all overlapping manifest dimensions out of *STEM.*

The edge of the *Mandelbrot set* through which fractals are formed is an abstract mathematical extrapolation of this final membrane. The singularity of a black hole is a point or spot on this last interface edge membrane. It is a trans-dimensional gate or portal. The push pull, *out-flow, in-flow,* expansion and contraction can be observed and verified throughout all layers and aspects of *STEM.* Outside *STEM* these polarized qualities cease to exist. As confirmation of the presence of *gravity waves* is verified, this may be the first step in substantiating these concepts.

Chaotic inflation asks: what came before the singularity that was the *Big Bang?* Many scientists suggest that this is a meaningless question, since *space-time* only sprang into existence with the advent of the *Big Bang.*

If time did not exist yet, then there was no before. The *chaotic inflation* theorists answer by suggesting that the universe came into existence through a *quantum fluctuation* from a *pre-existing* region of *space-time.*

This is the *budding universe* theory that speculates that from one *pre-existing space-time* physical universe, *quantum fluctuations* passed through a black hole singularity to make the *space-time* physical universe we live in. As this *process* is repeated over and over we have the *budding universe* or *multiverse.* In this model there is a before and an after. This theory generates a self-perpetuating infinite loop. This type of theoretical model is developed from and bound within *space-time.* That which is formulated in *space-time,* having *form,* cannot effectively describe or explain that which is beyond *space-time.* It can lead us to the edge of the last membrane having *form* and can be a bridge into the *formless.*

In this *inflationary cosmology,* I equate the *cosmologic constant* as a synonym for *quantum fluctuations, density fluctuations and density* or *primordial perturbations.* I believe all of these are terms identifying the presence and influence of gravity as it passes from the extra-dimensional *un-manifest no-thing* realm through the singularity of black holes into the manifest physical universe.

As this *quantum fluctuation, gravity vacuum* passes through the singularity of black holes into the manifest universe, it does not come from a *pre-existing* region of *space-time* constrained physical universe. It is, however, coming from a different dimension, devoid of any properties or characteristics of *space-time.*

The theoretical model that allows for *pre-existing* regions of *space-time* is what generates the conceptualization of a *multiverse*. The *multiverse* then allows for an unlimited number of parallel universes to exist.

This popular idea is being widely disseminated through all social media. TV shows often depict very entertaining CGI; computer generated imagery of the *multiverse.*

With *inflation,* the expanding balloon of the universe generates three primary options of what may happen in the future. First, it will expand forever. In this model, over time, everything will get further and further apart from each other as *space-time* becomes more and more dilute. Eventually, even the light of celestial objects will no longer be visible or traceable from or to each other. The observable universe will become totally black. This is the *vanishing universe model.* Currently there is a growing body of scientific research to support this theory.

A major component of this research is based on the fact that there is only about 23% of the necessary matter in the universe to account for the critical density required to explain gravitational effects on a universal scale. A *cosmologic constant,* as an abstract number or mathematical symbol, is introduced in an equation to account for the remaining critical density. The abstract *cosmologic constant* that validates *inflation* under these circumstances also demonstrates that the universe is spatially flat to within a few percentage points. In this model, the equations with the *cosmologic constant* added show that there is no point at which universal expansion will decelerate, therefore, it will expand forever.

The *cosmologic constant* is a purely theoretical mathematical abstraction, created to solve a previously unsolvable equation. This is a convenient expedient used by scientists as a rational conjecture.

If the number, added to solve the equation for inflation, coincidentally proving a flat universe, is inaccurate, then the conclusion of flatness is erroneous. Is there a *cosmologic constant* that still solves the equation for *inflation* but does not make the universe flat? This is the case in both the second and third options of future possibility.

The second option, is that the bubble or balloon of the universe will explode or pop. If it pops, this supports the concept of the *multiverse,* derived from a self-perpetuating loop and pop of *pre-existing space-times.* Although this theory is intriguing and garnering support, I suggest it makes for better science fiction than credible science.

The third option is that the expanding universe will stop expanding and start a cycle of contraction. This option is reflected from the microcosm to the macrocosm. At the beginning of this book I introduced the concept of cycles and the properties of a polarized universe. The dominant property of expansion and contraction in its many and varied *forms* has been demonstrated and extrapolated many times over. Everything in *STEM* has a beginning, with an expanding, growing, maturing *process.* At some linear point the expansion stops and contraction takes over as things shrink, age and die. Everything in *STEM* has a beginning and an end. This contracting model is known as the *big crunch.*

Einstein recognized all three of these possibilities. He found them all extremely disturbing, as did his colleagues. To neutralize these three options, Einstein added a *cosmologic constant* to his *general relativity equations* to create a stagnant, static and stable universe. Although Einstein's artificial abstraction, induction of a static universe was somewhat comforting, this comfort was shattered as proof of the expanding universe was realized. The most significant evidence of this expansion, is the *red shift*.

The *red shift* is an observation in astrophysics that as we look out into space, in every direction we see a displacement of the color spectrum emitted from every star and galaxy toward longer wavelengths. These longer wavelengths come from the red end of the spectrum and are caused as celestial objects move away from Earth.

The *quantum fluctuation, gravity vacuum, cosmologic constant* of *inflation* theory coming from another dimension, which is differentiated by different frequency or vibratory rates that are *un-manifest,* can neither be fully explained nor understood from a linear, mind derived construct dependent on the presence of *STEM; space-time,* energy and matter.

This presents a serious problem for science and scientists, as their methodology and tools will never be able to resolve this issue, unless by analogy they are willing to paint from a larger palette with more colors than were previously known or available. The ability to step out of the perceptual box of awareness and dearly held beliefs, and look back with a totally *unconditional* gaze through our *mind's eye,* is an act of creative imagination.

Development of this ability through diligent practice is essential. This is a tool of *spiritual technology* or *causation mechanics.*

Universal *Isotropy* and *Homogeneity* is a Reflection of *Source* Holographic Fragmentation

The *isotropic* and *homogeneous* character of the physical universe is a reflection of the inherent properties and characteristics of the holographic fragmentation of *source* essence as *Chi* spirit manifested *STEM.*

I suspect that *Inflation* is not so much the cause of the *isotropy* and *homogeneity* of the universe but rather an *effect* of the holographic fragmentation *process* of manifestation.

Each fragment is a miniature replica of the original *source* hologram. As these fragments expanded to make up the known universe, the qualities of *isotropy* and *homogeneity* became an inherent part of *STEM.*

It is fundamentally the holographic quality of existence that causes the *microcosm* and *macrocosm* to be mirror reflections of each other. The spiritual principles of *as-above - so-below* and *as-within - so-without* are also reflections of this holographic characteristic; from the inner worlds of the *un-manifest* to the outer worlds of the manifest and back again.

As the theory of the presence of *gravity waves* is realized and replicated, another small piece of the ineffable story of existence continues to unfold. I predict that as we develop the ability to consistently find and quantify gravity waves that we will discover that they have the same *homogeneity* throughout the universe as the background microwave radiation.

Einstein inserted a *cosmologic constant*, equal to the energy density of the vacuum of space into his *General Relativity field equations* to artificially induce a static model of the universe. His *cosmologic constant*, presumed to be equal to the energy density of the vacuum of space, was an attempt to neutralize seemingly extraneous gravitational effects throughout the universe.

His equations, without the *cosmologic constant*, support a model of the universe as expanding and eventually contracting. The equilibrium of a presumed static universe has been shown mathematically to be fundamentally unstable. This means that Einstein's *cosmologic constant* never actually demonstrated a static universe.

If the *cosmologic constant*, vacuum energy density used in *inflation* is a positive number, the negative pressure caused by it induces the accelerating *homogenous* expansion of *STEM*, postulated by *inflation theorists*.

Although gravity is expressed in the physical universe as small quantum fluctuations due to the physical gravitational effects of celestial bodies on each other, I believe that these effects pale relative to the effect of interstellar background *gravitational waves*.

One of the fundamental problems in modern physics is the inability to reconcile the gravitational effects observed in the universe. If gravity is indeed caused by objects having mass that warp the fabric of *space-time*, as Einstein would have us believe, then the problem is that there isn't enough matter in the universe to explain what gravity is doing.

Physicists are generally creative people with vivid imaginations from which they generate theories of how the universe works. The framework for their flights of fancy are linked to the scientifically based or proven foundation of the best science of the time.

Einstein's body of work and theory represents just such a foundation. The level of stability of such a foundation is very strong.

The ability to step outside that foundation and look back *unconditionally* is hard to achieve under the best of circumstances. It is even harder for those with very strong mental linear constructs of reality or existence.

It has been said, and demonstrated historically, that many of the greatest breakthroughs in science, rather than coming from the leaders of the status quo, come from outside that most prestigious and respected bastion of authority. Einstein himself represented just such an outsider, and over time, despite rejection and ridicule, changed the very core of our belief and understanding of the universe as we know it.

Is it time for another shift or expansion? Given the framework of *General Relativity,* the fundamental problem of the universe not having enough matter to explain gravitational influence has caused physicists to wax philosophical and theorize the presence of *dark matter* and *dark energy.* This simple and elegant solution is unusually convenient. Anytime what's happening in the universe can't be explained, by adding just the right amount of *dark matter* and *energy* into the equations, voilà, like magic, everything works out.

In this case, the *cosmologic constant* is derived from the theoretical amount of *dark energy* needed to make *General Relativity* still work.

We are prone to take what we believe is science fact and add seeming rational science conjecture to fill in the missing pieces of our understanding. With increasing data and research we either increase or decrease the probability and validity of our theories. Currently there is no substantial scientific evidence that either *dark matter* or *energy* exist.

In the beginning of this book I shared the idea that physical matter has extremely low density. Remember my example of squeezing planet Earth into a solid ball of matter? First, I suggested that it would be no larger than a baseball, then I suggested that this would be a gross exaggeration of size, if the *Big Bang* were true and all *space-time* sprang from an infinitesimally small speck.

Matter is mostly empty space. Given this fact, how much gravitational force is its mass capable of producing? To generate the gravitational influence necessary to maintain this universe, the amount of *dark matter* would be several times greater than all regular matter derived from all known celestial bodies, including black holes. I suspect that adequate evidence to support *dark matter* and *dark energy* as a viable solution to this gravity problem will not be found.

Any Number Consecutively Divided In Half Can Never Reach Zero

Let's revisit black holes. Physicists suggest that a black hole is created as a star collapses upon itself. First the aging star goes through a period of expansion. There is a critical point at which the mass of the expanding star induces a *presumed* gravity field greater than the pressure wave of its expansion. In the case of a *supernova* this induces a rapid reversal of the star from its expansion mode into a contraction mode.

This is *RI; reverse inflation.* The star contracts until its gravity is so great that it creates a black hole singularity, with so much gravity that all matter, light, *space* and *time* reaching its *event horizon* is sucked into it. Once the threshold of the *event horizon* is crossed, there is no turning back.

Accelerating from the *event horizon* to the singularity, time is compressed like an accordion pleat. This is a *harmonic progression.* Using music as an analogy, we go from an initial or fundamental tone to a half tone, third tone, quarter tone and beyond. In a black hole, a fundamental foundational, linear time reference point slows down in a harmonic sequence as it approaches the singularity. Through each *harmonic progression,* time slows down more and more.

In mathematics, any number divided in half, over and over, will never reach zero. At first, the division *process* causes the number to approach zero at lightning speed.

The proximity to zero is so close, so fast that it seems justifiable for all inherent and practical purposes, to ignore the tiny and insignificant anomaly approaching zero and concede the answer is zero. To make it cleaner mathematically, we introduce a number or abstract mathematical symbol that lets us always solve the equation to equal zero. Is it really any better or different whether we fudge a little and concede the answer is zero, or that we introduce an abstract number or symbol to accomplish the zero sum outcome?

As an analogy, the *cosmologic constant* used by Einstein and *inflation theorists,* to solve the anomalies of the physical universe, are exactly the same type of abstraction as that applied to the math problem of any number being divided in half.

Approaching the singularity of a black hole, time is *harmonically* compressed. It may seem as if we are being drawn into the singularity at faster than light speed. As we increase proximity to the singularity, although we get closer and closer, we can never quit reach it.

Physicists suggest that, under these circumstances, we and everything else that crosses the *event horizon* of a black hole are compressed against the edge of the singularity into a very dense contracted mass of matter with a very large gravitational field. These qualities are the same for all black holes.

An alternate perspective, in the context of the microcosm reflecting the macrocosm; *as-above - so-below* and *as-within - so-without,* can be observed from the nature and life cycle of a single dying star.

The dying star is a reflection; as a piece of the fractured hologram, of the nature and life cycle of the universe as a whole. A single star is a *form*. It has an edge or membrane. It is born, expands, then contracts and dies.

Stars with adequate mass have the potential to become black holes. Some stars contract and collapse over extended time intervals. A collapsing *supernova,* on the other hand, *implodes* and then rebound explodes at light speed. Some of these become black holes and some neutron stars.

Superimposing a model of a dying *supernova* on a model of the universe, an intriguing picture emerges. First is the *Big Bang.* This was a beginning or birth. *STEM; space-time,* energy and matter were *formed* or manifested from *no-thing* in an instant. In this instant *source,* as a hologram, using its *cause substrate* spirit essence as sound, vibration and frequency, induced the first primordial black hole. As *source* passed through the singularity of this first primordial black hole using its sound spirit essence as its carrier wave, it fractured into all the particles that manifested as *STEM.*

Gravity Passing out of Black Holes Creates Mass as Matter, Matter does not Create Gravity, It is a Reflection of It

Current evidence is that the expansion of the universe is slightly accelerating. What is causing this to happen and why? Imagine that the universe is an inflating balloon.

Einstein's image of *space-time* as a fabric is very apropos. A fabric or balloon surface is an edge. An edge or surface is a *form*. A *form* has a distinct boundary. A boundary defines a clear limit. In this model the entire universe consisting of *STEM* is finite. Although the outermost edge or membrane of the universe may be as amorphous as any star, it remains finite. A star's surface is liquid and gaseous, having a very diffuse unclear edge; it essentially remains a constrained *form* that is also finite.

Given an expanding universe, we reviewed three optional future outcomes. One was expansion of a more and more dilute universe. In this model, the universe may or may not have an edge or membrane. If it does have a membrane its stretchability is unrestricted. This model supports the conceptualization of an unlimited and infinite universe.

The second option, is that the bubble or balloon of the universe expands until it explodes or pops. In this model, as the expanding universe pops, it creates a new universe. This gives rise to the *multiverse* and generation of many parallel universes. In this second model, the universe has a membrane that has an absolute limit of stretchability. This model supports the conceptualization of a limited and finite universe.

The third option, is that the bubble or balloon of the universe reaches a critical, terminal point of expansion then starts to contract. This model also supports the conceptualization of a limited and finite universe.

With a dying *supernova,* the expanding star has a shorter quicker phase of expansion, prior to a rapid phase of implosion, then explosion, ending as a neutron star or black hole.

This current physical universe is starting this shorter quicker phase of expansion. Gravity is homogeneously distributed throughout the fabric of the universe. It is linked by *gravity waves* through the original primordial black hole to the pre-existing field of gravity on the other side. Remember my analogy of gravity being like an iceberg. The tip of the iceberg of gravity is in the physical universe. It is reflected as objects with mass attract each other.

The majority of gravity is the body of the iceberg in the dimension of the *un-manifest, no-thing* realm. It is from this other dimension that it has its greatest influence in the physical universe.

The majority of *gravity waves* are not induced from the quantum fluctuations of the physical gravitational effects caused by celestial bodies attracting each other.

My conjecture is that the majority of *gravity waves* are either coming directly out of the singularities of black holes, or they manifest physically because of the continuous gravitational force being exerted from the *un-manifest, no-thing* dimensional gravity field on the other side of black holes. Imagine that these *gravity waves* are exerting a continuous gravitational pull on all of the physical universe as *STEM,* uniformly and consistently.

Consider the possibility that mass, as matter, is not the primary, primordial source of gravity. Before the *Big Bang* there was no *space-time* or matter.

Is it possible that the force of gravity pre-existed the *Big Bang* and the manifestation of *STEM*? Given this possibility, it may be that gravity is part of what causes mass and matter to give *form* increased physical density, not the other way around.

As this gravitational pull approaches, then supersedes a force equal to the force expanding the physical universe, there is a short rebound acceleration of the expansion of the physical universe before it starts to contract.

This acceleration, whether from an individual star or the universe at large, is a reflexive response of final resistance to the gravitational force of contraction pulling from the other side of a black hole. Once the accelerated expansion is overwhelmed by gravity, contraction starts. If the universe's contraction parallels the death of a *supernova* this initial contraction will be accelerated, a virtual *reverse inflation*.

RI; Reverse Inflation

Given the current accelerated expansion of the physical universe, how close in linear time, might *reverse inflation* start? Some physicists have speculated that this contraction will start in ten to twenty billion years.

In some spiritual and religious circles this contraction is imminent. This perspective is derived from some interpretations, of both Christian biblical references, as well as correlations of the *Mayan Calendar.* The destructive side of these references suggest that we are about to enter the end times and experience Armageddon. A rapid contraction, *RI; reverse inflation* event would support this option.

The constructive side of these same references suggest, rather than imminent destruction, we are on the cusp of a major cycle shift. This is a shift of awakening consciousness and remembering, an Earth mother, *Gaia* centered reemergence. Cooperation, tolerance, service and *unconditional* love will be the guiding principles of this shift.

An alternate timeline for the universe to start contraction, comes from the Hindu cycle of cosmic history called a *Mahayuga.* A *Mahayuga* consists of a *Satya Yuga* or *Golden Age,* lasting 1,728,000 years, a *Tretya Yuga* or *Silver Age* lasting 1,296,000 years, a *Dwapara Yuga* or *Copper Age* lasting 864,000 years and a *Kali Yuga* or *Iron Age* lasting 432,000 years.

The current *Kali Yuga* started around 3102 BC with the death of *Krishna.* This leaves approximately 427,000 years before the contraction of the universe either starts or will have ended.

When the cycle of a *Mahayuga* ends the entire physical universe is resorbed through the singularity of a black hole, back into the *un-manifest, no-thing* dimension from which it came.

After an equal amount of time, as a *Mahayuga*, the physical universe will manifest anew. This great cycle is identified as one day in the life of *Brahma; source* essence or God. This repeating cycle is to last for 100 *Brahma* years, equal to 311 trillion, 40 billion human years.

The purpose of this repeating cycle is for the particles of the fractured hologram that is *source* to wake up, to *be* self and then God realized. That which is manifest as a polarized dimension, is the training ground of *soul,* which is a unit of consciousness or particle from the ocean that is the *source* hologram. The cycle repeats and repeats, giving *soul* experiences within polarity to learn from and eventually master as *machaneers.* *Machaneers* are master engineers of *causation* or *process mechanics.* As *cause,* we are here to serve *unconditionally.*

We learn to give and receive divine love and to take our place as *conduits* of divine will. The essence of this is to wake up and take back control of our divine connection and show others how to do the same. Historically, in any given cycle, some *souls* make it through and some do not.

I hold the space that all have been chosen and the time is now. The purpose of the repeating cycles is to offer and allow *soul* another opportunity, through experiences, to wake up. If we don't get it, we are given the privilege to try again, until we do get it. When we do get it, then we can choose to stop participation in the cycle. If we choose to continue participation, we function as *machaneers,* this is an act of service.

Time Slows As A *Harmonic Progression*

As we approach the singularity of a black hole, time is slowed down, through a *harmonic progression.* At the singularity of a black hole, all matter, light, *space* and *time* pass through. They are not compressed against the surface of the singularity into a super dense mass of matter with an extremely large gravity field.

For consciousness to cross the final membrane between *STEM* and the *un-manifest, no-thing* dimension, there is no linear mind based tool or mechanism available to augment this crossing. As time slows to nothing, approaching the singularity of a black hole, the only way for consciousness to cross to the other side is to completely release *be-mi;* body, ego, mind and identity. This surrender can be enhanced and the transition potentiated by engaging *USL; universal sound language,* and achieving effective release and control of body *fascia.*

The natural state of body *fascia* is complete permeability. It is fundamentally permeable to two things; the sound current we call spirit or *Chi,* and consciousness. Every point of conscious contact on the fascial membrane is a Mandelbrot set or black hole singularity. Matter that is drawn back from whence it came, through a black hole singularity, ceases to exist. From *no-thing* came everything; then everything reverts back to the *un-manifest no-thing.* The essence of spirit and consciousness is not matter. They exist prior to and completely independently of *STEM.*

As spirit and consciousness are drawn back through the singularity of a black hole, they are neither destroyed nor cease to exist; they remain unscathed.

STEM is a training ground for *soul awakening.* All of *STEM* is impermanent, transitory and finite. The term *Maya,* derived from Eastern mysticism, roughly translated as illusion or delusion, is used to differentiate that which is real; yet impermanent, from that which is real; yet permanent or infinite. *STEM* is *Maya.* It is *soul* and spirit that are infinite. *STEM* is made manifest and goes through a cycle of expansion, then contraction. At its apex of contraction all *STEM* is sucked back into the void through the singularity of a black hole into nothingness.

The gravity field or *gravity waves* at the singularity of a black hole cannot continue to be generated from a mass of denser and denser contracted matter. Since all the matter gets sucked through into nothingness, the gravity field or *gravity waves* must be coming out of the black hole singularity itself. As an analogy; food is not the *source* of *Chi* or life force in the physical domain, but merely a carrier or conduit for it. So too is gravity not the *source* of *Chi* or life force but merely a carrier or conduit of spirit as well. Is it possible that a special and unique quality of gravity is its capacity to function as a carrier medium for spirit from the *unmanifest* to the manifest?

Dark Gravity Reflected As Gravity Waves Is the Cosmologic Constant

I suspect that the real *cosmologic constant* is primarily the gravity field emanating through the singularities of black holes as *gravity waves.* What pulls all the matter through is not gravity being induced as a star collapses on itself but the gravity field pulling the star from the other side of the black hole singularity. At the singularity of a black hole there is no matter and no actual gravity well. The black hole is a portal between dimensions. Through this portal all *STEM* is made manifest and all *STEM* returns *un-manifest, as in-flow* and *out-flow* on a universal scale. Imagine God pushing out with *HU* from itself, from the ocean of one that *IT IS.* God's voice creates and sustains all things, in all dimensions. *Out-flow* differentiates into polarity. Now imagine God pulls in with *HU* and draws back into itself all that is. This is God's breath.

The *cosmologic constant* is gravity in all its *forms.* Is it possible that as gravity enters the physical universe that its wave *form* repels, thus inducing an expanding universe? Is it possible that as gravity returns to its origin that its wave *form* attracts, inducing a contracting universe? Is it possible that the *cosmologic constant* is a variable figure? The *cosmologic constant* for expansion may be an inverse of the *cosmologic constant* for contraction.

Dark gravity is a theory that stipulates there is no additional energy density component in the universe. This makes *dark matter* and *dark energy* obsolete.

Is it possible that *dark gravity* may be reflected as *gravity waves* in the physical universe and these waves originate from and through the singularity of black holes? A fine tuning or revision of Einstein's *General Relativity* equations are probable indicated.

The New Scientific Method to Integrate Spiritual Technology and Traditional Science

An acceptable scientific proof in the manifest, material physical dimensions requires that the proof be objective and replicable by or from an external source.

The exact same experimental parameters must be utilized. Traditional science emphasizes externalized data and frequently is dependent on machine technology.

If science is to more fully understand the nature of our existence, purpose and meaning in life, in the broadest context, then traditional science must develop a segue to spiritual technology.

Traditional science is a reasonable approach and tool in the dimensions that range from the gross physical, through the emotional, to the mental. These are the dimensions of *space-time*.

These are the dimensions of causality; cause and effect, as well as polarity; positive and negative energy charge. It is these qualities which have allowed us to formulate and then apply our current model for scientific research and proof.

Since this method has proven itself over and over with practical and useful technologic advances for everyday use, it is easy to see how both the scientific and lay community has wholeheartedly adopted these methods as critical, essential and irreplaceable.

Applying the scientific method, constrained in its current *form* to explain or understand everything is neither practical nor possible. Although modern science is being utilized to conduct research on spiritual topics frameable in polarized dimensions, this same science is inadequate to the task of research outside *STEM.*

A broader definition or application of scientific method, to include what I frame as *spiritual technology* or *spiritual science*, is an essential adjunct as our awareness, perception and knowledge base expands on our journey upwards, inwards and beyond *STEM.*

In the *un-manifest, no-thing* dimensions, spiritual technology or science emphasizes internal subjective data versus external objective data. Spiritual technology or science is independent of any machine technology. To understand and explain gravity and other extra-dimensional influences, the integration of physical science and spiritual science is essential.

Acknowledging that a proof can be subjective and replicable from an internal *source*, utilizing similar but not exact experimental parameters is the first step.

Dimensions Overlap as Different Energy, Frquency and Vibrational States, not as Parallels

All the levels of *String Theory* are overlapping, not parallel. The levels theorized from *String Theory* can be extrapolated to the levels of perception applied to a physical pencil. As a pencil is perceived through our five physical senses, a microscope, the chemical-molecular level, atomic and sub-atomic levels, it is confirmed that these levels of differentiation overlap. This exemplifies the axiom; *as-above - so-below, as-within - so-without.*

Each level of perception or knowledge of the pencil is true and correct. These levels are not parallel but overlapping. No level negates another, nor is one more accurate than another, each is merely additive.

As each level is added, our perception and knowledge is expanded. From the contracted, to the expanded, to the more expanded; this is the *in-flow, out-flow* pulse wave of consciousness in action.

Each level offers a different, even radical, perception or awareness of an object or its properties. Each level is a description of the same thing. It is accurate to state that each level is, in a fundamental way, a reflection of every other level.

If this perspective is applied to both the *Quantum Physics* microcosm, which encompasses the world of the very small, atomic and sub-atomic particles, and to the *Relativity Theory* macrocosmic world of the very large, including the universe and all celestial bodies, then both systems are reflections of each other.

Neither negates the other; together they are merely additive. Based on the same fundamentals, it can be extrapolated; *Quantum Physics, Relativity Theory,* and now *String Theory,* can all be identified as reflections of each other. None of the three negate each other; together they are merely additive.

Quantum Mechanics, Relativity Theory, String Theory (Reconciled)

These reflective images are not like regular physically reflected images that are recognizable as the same thing, such as a reflection from a mirrored surface. From the *Quantum level*, in isolation, we are blind to the *Relativity level.* From the *Relativity level,* in isolation, we have the same blind spot effect. When we step beyond, or look back from the other side of a black hole singularity the reflections are in crystal clear focus.

The primary difference between these levels, is a function of frequency or vibration. From any given frequency vibrational level all other levels are invisible.

Throughout history, every time we believe, think or seemingly prove the nature of things or reality, we demonstrate the additive nature of our awareness, understanding and perceptual foundation.

An example is the electro-magnetic field. The first level of awareness and perception of the electro-magnetic field is personal direct experience of the visible spectrum of light. In the year 1800, the infrared level of the electro-magnetic spectrum was identified, and the concept of the spectrum itself was recognized. Both visible light and infrared are different band widths of the same fundamental wave *form.*

In the 1900's, the purported full spectrum of electro-magnetism was identified, with the discovery of gamma rays. The electro-magnetic spectrum ranges between radio waves at one end and gamma rays at the other.

In the broader context of this spectrum, we know and understand that visible light only represents an extremely small portion of the full spectrum. Due to our awakening awareness of the additive and expanded principle of the nature of awareness, knowledge, understanding and perception, scientists have speculated that the actual electro-magnetic spectrum is probably infinite and continuous.

Hu-man Advanced Civilizations on Planet Earth may Pre-Date Previous Theory

There is a growing body of archeological evidence that our historical perspective on the emergence of early man on the planet and the development of more advanced civilizations may be inaccurate.

Some evidence points to more advanced civilizations both pre-dating and parallel in time, with primitive earlier developmental stages of modern humans. Theories of Atlantis and Lemuria support this historical premise. More relevant than these theories is new archeological data coming from numerous dig sites.

Gregg Braden in his latest book, *Deep Truth,* identifies several archeological sites that pre-date the known historical emergence of more advanced human civilizations.

The ages of more advanced civilizations previously believed to have started with Sumer and Egypt approximately 5,000 years ago are being superseded. From Caral in Peru at 5,000 to 7,000 years old, to the Gulf of Khambhat in India at 9,500 years old, to Gobekli Tepe in Turkey at 9,000 to 11,000 years old. Finds at these sites demonstrate advances in art, science, math and architecture and no evidence of weapons or other signs of war or violence.

All the archeological sites from Sumer to the present have weapons and clear signs of war. Is it possible that the current prevailing paradigm of humans *being* a warring species is not an accurate reflection of what Braden would call a *Deeper Truth?* He suggests that the authentic nature of humans is one of cooperation rather than violent competition.

Indigenous people in their oral histories share stories and mythology of cycles reflected as *great world ages.* Braden correlates these ages to cycles of climate change and postulates the ebb and flow of war and violence being linked to these cycles.

He claims that we are on the cusp bridging the 5th to the 6th world age. This transition not only represents a 5,000 year interval between individual ages but also represents the transition of a larger cycle of 25,000 years between each of five world ages combined.

These 5,000 and 25,000 year cycles are part of a pattern of cycles that are smaller and larger than either of these, as reflected in the cycle of a *Mahayuga*. This supports our natural progression from a contracted; less than knowledge base, to an expanded; greater than knowledge base.

This *process* moves back and forth in a repeating cycle between expansion and contraction. This is the time of the *Great Awakening and Remembering.*

What to expect after *RST:* Resonant Sound Therapy

A common reaction after an *RST* session is to experience an increase in sensory acuteness, clarity or intensity. Feelings are often more pronounced. Both laughing and crying may surface more frequently and easily.

If a treatment session includes cranial contact, the patient may experience an increased awareness and intensity of dreams. They may also be aware of more visual and auditory perception or presence. Colors or sounds may seem brighter or clearer. This perception or presence is often apparent whether one's eyes are open or closed, whether in a quiet place or not. Blue is one of the dominant colors that people visualize. It may have a pulsing or spiraling quality.

Patients also report more clicking, popping and electronic or humming sounds. They may mistake these sounds as tinnitus or ringing sounds in the ears. Tinnitus is usually caused by a mechanical or nerve related injury. The sounds induced with *RST* are the result of a *tuning* mechanism establishing a wider band-width of perception.

As Hu-mans, we are transmitters and receivers. The perception or belief that we are limited by the range or band-width of our five primary senses of sight, sound, smell, taste and touch is self-induced.

This limited perceptual range is re-enforced through our body and mind linkage to our linguistic, familial, social, cultural, religious and political up-bringing and indoctrination. The decrease in perceptual band-width is a consequence of *being* out of calibration.

RST is a system, tool or technique to re-establish our normal and full calibration potential. As we calibrate, the clicking, popping, electronic or humming sounds progress into sounds heard in nature, like running water, wind, the ocean, bees or the sound of a flute. They may also develop into music, either simple or as complex as full symphonies.

If you relax and let yourself follow the light or visual images, as well as the sound, you may be surprised and pleased with the results.

7 Self-Help, Home Activities

A major factor in the significant increase in auto-immune disease, mental illness and other physical, emotional, mental and spiritual imbalances is our energetic physical disconnection with Earth.

I present my patients with a seven item self-help hand-out after their first *RST* session.

1. After *RST* drink lots of pure water. Use tested and certified pure spring or well water. Tap water is an option too, with additional filtration using a solid carbon-block with .02 micron filtration or reverse osmosis. I do not recommend distilled water. Although it is purified, it is energetically inert. The life force, or *Chi,* is radically reduced.

Short term, modest use of distilled water is acceptable, but frequent or continuous use will be de-stabilizing. Water should neither be transported, stored nor used from plastic containers regardless of claims of purity, benefit or safety.

PH modified water, at a minimum of 7.0 or higher significantly increases the body's ability to hold fluid in cells. Loss of intra-cellular fluid is a major component of disease induction and aging.

Structuring water is ancient. Modern applications essentially recognize that water passed through any structure that induces a spiraling or helical influence increases *Chi* and energetic equilibrium. Water is the *staff* of life, a universal solvent and detoxicant.

Without adequate water, equilibrium is compromised in the body and in anything else that can be an ally for our health, well-*being* and *awakening*.

I suggest one eight ounce glass of pure water per hour, or more if engaging vigorous exercise or sweating. Reduce consumption as evening or bedtime approaches, unless you want to have a disturbed sleep cycle, due to increased urination.

2. Daily *grounding*, establishes and maintains our essential connection with the energy field, or *Chi* of the planet. Ideally this is done barefoot, standing on dirt, sand, grass, gravel, soil or rock. A slightly reduced connection can be established standing inside on wood or tiles made from ceramic, marble, brick or slate.

One-hundred percent wool carpet or rugs increases the field. Laminate flooring, as long as the primary material occurs in nature, is adequate.

For any of these natural materials to be adequately *grounded,* part of their edge must reach the edge of the building foundation. This allows the planet's energy field to arc from Earth, over the concrete slab, through the natural material of the floor covering. A simple concrete slab, due to its composition and density, painted or not, has a dampening or reducing effect. Synthetic carpets or other completely synthetic materials, block the Earth's field even more.

Synthetic socks should not be used. Cotton, wool or a cotton wool blend sock is best. Wear a one-hundred percent leather bottom moccasin, optimally with barefeet. The outside surface of the moccasin must be in physical contact with any naturally *grounded* material, whether indoors or outdoors.

Until the leather of a moccasin has been broken in, by continuous movement and contact with *grounded* materials, its permeability to the Earth's field is diminished. Any other natural foot wear, like woven grass sandals or wooden clogs also work. Socks may be worn with moccasins or other natural foot wear but are not ideal. The Earth's energy field, or *Chi* band-width, is not limited exclusively within, or derived from the known electro-magnetic spectrum.

The implication that non-electrically *grounded* materials, like wood, are not good *grounding* surfaces represents a limited view or perception of what actually constitutes *grounding. Grounding* is much more than a connection with the electro-magnetic portion of Earth's energy-*Chi* field.

3. To engage the first three position, movements of *Resonant Movement Meditation (RMM)*. *Being grounded*, although healthy and balancing, is not, in itself, adequate to maintain optimal health and *well-being*. It is the potentiation and magnification of Earth's essential life force *Chi in-flow*, as well as the *Cosmic Universal, Trans-Dimensional Chi out-flow* that is critical for consistently maintainable energetic balance, health and *well-being*.

Both *RMM and RST* function to potentiate and magnify *Chi* flowing in and out of the physical body. Ideally, these first three positions of *RMM* and the addition of number four should be done for about a half hour daily. When that much time is not available, any time interval, including a couple of minutes, can bring significant results. I often find myself squeezing in two minute sessions several times daily.

When starting, identify and orient yourself to one of the four cardinal directions of the compass. This is to start to reestablish your sacred connections. Open your heart, *be unconditional,* invite *Earth Mother,* all her *spirits* and *divine, source, God* to connect with and guide you. Ideally, wear natural fiber clothing and remove all metal jewelry surrounding any part of the body. Empty your pockets, remove cell phones and watches.

Position One: *Individuation;* While *grounded,* stand up straight with your arms relaxed, hanging by your sides. Place your feet approximately one foot width wider than your shoulders, toes facing forward. Bounce from your knees; now lightly clench and unclench your hands in synchronous rhythm with your bouncing.

Close your eyes and *tone HU. HU* is a reference starting tone. It is a *mantra. Mantras* are syllables of *USL;* the *Universal Sound Language. USL* is embedded in, and is an integral part, of all languages. *USL* is found in all religious and spiritual teachings.

Toning may utilize or integrate any vocal sound or combination of sounds. The range, pitch and volume of vocal sound is individualized and variable. *Toning* may use vowel sounds, like A, E, I, O and U or any of numerous *mantras*, which include Aum, Baju, Hum or *HU. Toning*, whether being used personally, as *RMM* or with a therapist as *RST,* may also integrate singing songs with uplifting lyrics, playing music or using drums, bells, bowels or anything to augment *toning* during sessions.

Modulate personal amplitude and frequency to optimize *Chi* connection. This is the *individuation process*, inherent in *RST and RMM.* Modulation is change.

The amplitude is the depth of your knee bend; the smaller the bend, the lower the amplitude. The frequency is the speed of your bounce; slower is a lower frequency, faster is a higher frequency.

If unable to stand, the basic principles of shaking the body with *toning* can be implemented sitting in a chair, in a bed or on the floor. This applies to any of the following positions. Simple singing and dancing are essentially basic *forms* of *RMM.*

Any singing is *toning* and any dancing involves rhythmic circular, rotational motion. To emulate *RMM,* engage singing and dancing while *grounded* to the Earth.

Position Two-A: *In-flow;* while *grounded,* stand up straight. Place your feet approximately one foot width wider than your shoulders, toes facing forward. Bend your knees just enough to feel your feet spread and flatten. Hold your arms from shoulder to elbows pressed against your sides. Bend your elbows, so your forearms are at a 90 degree angle from your body, with your hands facing palms up.

Stretch the hands so they are flat, or even convex. Make a *counter-clockwise* circular rotation from the hips only, while *toning*. This opens a channel for Earth's life force *Chi* to pass through the body as a spiral, from the outside-in and the bottom-up.

Earth *Chi* flows through the acupuncture point *kidney one;* the bubbling well spring, on the bottom of the feet, up through all the meridians and *chakras.* This is *in-flow;* one half of the *double helical form* of *Chi* as it moves from the manifest, polarized dimensions inwardly, across the *membrane* that divides it from the *un-manifest, no-thing* dimensions out of *space-time* and matter.

Position Two-B: *Out-flow;* Replicate Position Two-A, but now make a *clockwise* circular rotation, from the hips only, while *toning.* This opens a channel for inner dimensional Universal Cosmic *Chi.* This *Chi* passes through the body as a spiral, from the inside-out and the top-down.

This is *out-flow;* the other half of the *double helical form* of *Chi,* as it moves from the *un-manifest, no-thing* dimensions across the *membrane* that divides it from the manifest dimensions into *space-time* and matter.

<u>Position Three</u>: *Mobius*: while *grounded* and *toning,* combine the *counter-clockwise* and *clockwise* circles of <u>Position Two-A and B</u> into a figure eight twisted in three dimensions. This is a *mobius,* which is an infinity symbol. It increases the magnitude of *Chi* flowing through the body. The initial *Chi* entering *space-time* that is devoid of dimensionality becomes one, then quickly, two dimensional, as the *counter-clockwise in-flow* and *clockwise out-flow* circles of *Chi* overlap in *space-time,* forming a spiral figure eight.

Chi, in-flowing and *out-flowing,* as a spiral figure eight, hits the membrane edge of *fascia* surrounding and encapsulating every part of the body simultaneously. As the two dimensional spiral figure eight hits fascial membranes, it warps and twists, becoming three dimensional. This three dimensional quality, induced as *Chi* hits the first physically manifest fascial membrane, is a *mobius.* As the *mobius* passes through *fascia,* its spiral tightens, becoming a *double helix.* Energetically balanced *Chi,* in the *form* of the *double helix,* passing through *fascia,* un-winds and releases the torque or twist of *fascial* membranes caused by physical, emotional and mental injury or trauma, as well as mental projection judgments. This release allows *Chi* to flow without restriction throughout all body *fascia.*

Acupuncture Meridians and *Chakras* exist physically in body *fascia.* They are zones of increased or concentrated *Chi* flow layered in fascial sheets. The physical and functional relationship between *fascia* and meridians gives a clear scientific basis as to why and how acupuncture works.

Unwound *fascia* with unrestricted *Chi* flow induces energetic equilibrium. This is a balance between *in-flow* and *out-flow.* This brings *healing* and well-*being* to *mind-body* and *spirit.* Consistently moving energetically balanced *Chi,* as an *in-flow and out-flow* through the body, over-rides *Newton's Third Law* of *Motion,* which states that for every action there is an equal and opposite reaction; known as the law of *cause* and *effect.* This allows us to *transcend,* thereby suspending the *action-reaction* operation of *cause* and *effect,* to *be cause* and control our destiny.

While *grounded, toning and* physically moving in the *counter-clockwise* and *clockwise* spirals that *form* a *mobius,* a release is initiated from the pull of the *downward spiral* that sustains and maintains life as effect.

The necessary commitment to personally actualize Position One, Two and Three, gives us a subjective, experiential basis to *feel Chi* as it passes through the body. The ability to consistently *feel Chi,* places us on the *inward-upward expanding spiral* that sustains and maintains life as *cause.*

The ability to differentiate whether we are moving up or down the spiral, and then choosing our direction, is a critical step in our *healing* and *awakening journey.* Be mindful and observant, and notice if there is any subjective sensation you can feel in the palms of your hands as you do <u>Position Three</u>. This sensation is a direct experience of *Chi* moving through the body.

The actual feeling of this energy sensation is the beginning of the induction of an energy equilibrium state in the body that brings balance, healing and increased awareness. One of the characteristics of body *Chi* sensation is tingling. If you are feeling anxious, tired, have physical pain or are depressed, even short intervals of these position movements can offer amazing and quick relief. When possible, fifteen to thirty minute sessions are recommended.

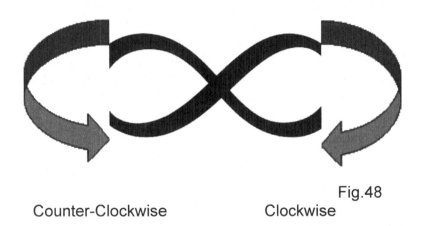

Fig.48

Counter-Clockwise   Clockwise

4A. While standing, *grounded* and *toning,* alternate using open hands and closed fists, to hit yourself from the top of your collar bones, to as far as your arms reach down the front of your legs. Continue alternating open hands and closed fists as you hit the sides of your legs, then your buttocks. Start with *AH* as your vocal sound. Repeat, going from the top-down and the bottom-up several times. This can be done with a light, to forceful touch, a loud or soft voice.

Balanced rhythmic beating is a remarkable tool to help us awaken and release *fascia.* This is more effective if *grounded* but can be done anywhere, anytime.

If you can only do this with rubber soled shoes on synthetic carpet in a multi-storied metal framed building, do it anyway. If you have the opportunity to do this exercise *grounded* and not *grounded,* can you feel the difference?

4B. Stand *grounded* and *toning.* Hit your right fist or open hand to your left thigh while at the same time hitting your right buttock with your left fist or open hand. Rotate your body as you do this so that you're swinging arms and swinging torso hit each other in opposite directions. Swing and rotate your body to the right, *clockwise* as your right arm is swinging to the left, *counterclockwise.*

Reverse the body swing to the left and both arms and hands to the right. Work your way up to your collarbones and over your back and then back down again. Do not hurt yourself. Hit, twist and stretch within the constraints of your own body limits.

With time, diligence and care, you will get stronger and more flexible. Remember the adage; *use it or lose it.*

If weak or debilitated, or as an alternate to 4B, while lying on your back, on any surface with your legs slightly apart, bring your large toes together, then apart. Keep your legs down on the flat surface. Try to create a forty-five degree angle or more, both turning inward as well as outward. Do this at any speed. You can also alternate the in-out motion with an up-down motion.

This is to flex your feet toward your head, then extend them down. These motions emulate and activate both the spiral of the figure eight and the helix. This also induces a *cross-crawl,* which is the way infants learn to crawl prior to walking. This repairs and re-establishes a balanced feedback between the central and peripheral nervous systems.

It is a powerful tool for stroke patients or other neurologically compromised conditions. There is a mechanical machine called the *Chi machine* that does this passively for a patient.

5. Ideally, everything that goes into the mouth should be smelled first, including water. Smell individual items with your eyes closed. Be sure that you can identify the item correctly, based on smell exclusively, without a visual reference counter-point. Practice and learn to trust smell as a determinant to guide you as to whether to put the item into your mouth or body. The *olfactory bulb* transmits smell signals to the brain for processing. The *olfactory bulb* is the tip of the *limbic system.* This system in the middle of the brain, is the master control center for all neuro-endocrinologic functions, emotional equilibrium and it influences autonomic nervous system function and balance.

Smell, and the re-establishment of its proper use and function, is a remarkable and powerful ally in our personal journey of health, *well-being* and *enlightenment.* With a complex food mixture, smell the bouquet and try to isolate as many individual ingredients as possible. We should even smell our medications and supplements. Be grateful and mindful.

When possible, eat while *grounded*. Eat with your hands or wooden chopsticks, wood or ceramic utensils. Bamboo-ware is available from my web-site or clinic. Try to avoid or minimize metal utensils.

Most metal, being electro-conductive, creates a warping of *Chi* transmission from food through the silverware into the body. This potentiates food allergies and other auto-immune imbalances.

Chew food until it is liquid. *Be* mindful and grateful, chew each bite, feel the texture with teeth and tongue. As fiber and muscle break up under the pressure of our teeth, a portion of the bite becomes liquid and we swallow it. Continue chewing as more of the bite liquefies and swallow again. Continue this process with each bite until it has been liquefied and swallowed. This may represent as many as seventy chews. Practice counting to compare the different texture and density of foods. You may find yourself spontaneously being drawn to place another mouthful of food into your mouth before the last part of the last bite is fully chewed and swallowed.

This common behavior reflex affords the opportunity to practice *circular eating*; following the principle of chewing and continuously swallowing only that portion of any given bite that is liquid. This is a parallel to what is called *circular breathing,* an essential skill for playing the *didgeridoo*. This is a type of *pranayama,* which is controlled *yogic* slow breathing. This is an important tool of *causation mechanics* and *enlightenment.*

Slowing down, allows us to tangibly feel life force *Chi* transmitted from food into the body. Life force *Chi* sustains and nourishes, a truly wonderful and delightful experience. Vitamins, minerals, protein, carbohydrate and enzymes are physical dimension shell membrane *forms* to encapsulate life essence. They are not the *source* of *Chi* but carriers of it.

Apply the 80-20 rule. Follow these guidelines 80% of the time or more, if possible. Practice moderation in all things. It's not what we do occasionally that harms us, but what we do all the time.

6. Do self or shared *Foot Reflexology* daily. This is simply foot massage. Add *toning.* The *blue-print* of the body is on the surface and bottom of the feet. This is literal not hypothetical. All terminal branches of *fascia* end on the feet.

Massage the foot from the top of the ankles over the entire foot, including the top, sides, between the toes and bottom. Twist, pull, push and press every part. This can be done with either light or hard pressure. Don't be shy, push your tolerance range.

As *fascia* is released on the feet, it releases everywhere in the body. *Fascia* is *contiguous;* connected everywhere.

Looking at a reflexology chart of the body part correlations, reflexed over the surface and bottom of the foot, is unnecessary, although educational.

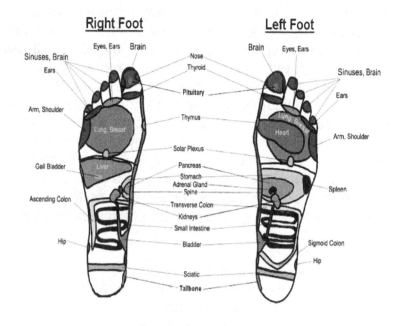

Right Foot | **Left Foot**

Eyes, Ears Brain Nose
Sinuses, Brain Thyroid
Ears Pituitary
Arm, Shoulder Thymus
Lung, Breast Solar Plexus
Gall Bladder Liver Pancreas
Stomach
Adrenal Gland
Ascending Colon Spine
Transverse Colon
Kidneys
Small Intestine
Hip Bladder
Sciatic
Tailbone

Brain Eyes, Ears
Sinuses, Brain
Ears
Lung, Breast Arm, Shoulder
Heart
Spleen
Sigmoid Colon
Hip

Fig. 49

FOOT REFLEXOLOGY CHART

7. *RST* sessions induce the *Homeopathic* principle of *retracing*; which states that *healing* occurs from the inside-out and from the top-down, with physical, emotional or mental symptoms, manifesting in the reverse order of their occurrence in our *life-existence*. This *retracing* can be mild, to severe. *Retracing* is a natural and unavoidable consequence of un-winding the fascial membrane. *Fascia* holds, then releases, the negative energetic charge induced from physical injury, or any experience, memory or image-projection linked with any negatively charged emotion like fear, anger, sadness, pain, lust, greed, vanity or attachment.

Fascia also holds and releases any mental projections as judgments of guilt, shame or blame. Commonly, this *retracing* response occurs during day one to three after a treatment session. Since everyone is unique, *retracing* may occur at differing time intervals which may be significantly longer than three days, watch for this. *Retracing* is a real-time replay and release of physical, emotional or mental energy-*engram* patterns embedded in the fascial membrane. The *engram* is a stored memory trace or *recording* of a past traumatic or painful event that has occurred at some linear point in our *existence. Engrams* may be conscious or unconscious.

With RST, retracing is not only from the inside-out and top-down, but simultaneously from the bottom-up and the outside-in. This is a function of the dual spirals of Earth *Chi*, bringing *in-flow,* and the Cosmic *Chi*, bringing *out-flow.* It is the contact and passing through *fascia* of the *in-flow, out-flow* of *Chi,* as the *double helix* that unwinds fascial twisting.

It is twisted *fascia* that holds energy-*engram* patterns. Unwinding fascial twisting releases *engrams.* Releasing *engrams* is *retracing. RST* activates both aspects of the double helix of *Chi* flowing through the body. It is rhythmic clockwise rotational touch with *toning* that induces *retracing* from the inside-out and the top-down.

It is rhythmic counter-clockwise rotational touch with *toning* that induces *retracing* from the bottom-up and the outside-in. This aspect of *retracing* is potentiated when a therapist is *grounded* to the Earth, using applications of *pure essential oils.* These oils activate the *limbic system,* which is primarily influenced by smell.

The *limbic system* is the master control center for all neuro-endocrinologic functions. It influences the autonomic nervous system functions, and is the site of the body's emotional core.

It is *critically important*, when any *retracing* occurs, to *be* mindful and observant. *Retracing* that causes an increase or reactivation of old physical, emotional and mental injuries or traumas can be destabilizing and drive us into a negative feedback loop. To avoid this, be pro-active, quickly and actively engage the seven self-help principles.

This *process* of *in-flow* and *out-flow, contraction* and *expansion, decrease and increase* of symptoms, is both inevitable and unavoidable. The *retracing process* is the inherent action in all authentic *healing.*

A *retracing* exercise:

Play a movie picture of your life, from your birth forward. As you play this movie, carefully watch for any images with any negative emotional content or judgment.

When this occurs, it is usually overtly uncomfortable and may have distinct negative body sensations associated with it. This may be a headache or feeling of pressure in the head, tightness or a feeling of pressure or stress in the neck, shoulders, chest or belly. These body sensations are not limited to the aforementioned locations. Often we are directed to avoid, deny or suppress any of these images, feelings or body symptoms.

The consequence of engaging suppression or denial deepens and prolongs the very things we are attempting to avoid. These same images, feelings, judgments and body sensations also occur spontaneously, without intentional review of life experiences. The images come from our own conscious or subconscious minds and are either memories or projections of possible futures.

We create, share, read and watch external images through stories, books, TV and movies. We are also potentially capable, as well, of linking these non-personal external images with negatively charged emotions and or mental projection judgments.

In any of these cases:

Freeze frame the specific charged image. Stop it and hold it.

Next, loop it. Cut the specific scene out of your life movie or spontaneous experience, memory, projection, book, TV show or movie and then, play it over and over. Identify the negative emotional hooks and/or mental projection judgments associated with any specific image or body symptom.

As an exercise in creative imagination, take the hooks out. Take the fear, sadness, anger or pain, as well as any other negative feelings or mental judgment projections out of the looping scene. Imagine them as energetic non-physical hooks, knifes, spears, arrows, swords or bullets.

As this is done, our mind or body may be screaming to us that the pain, both physical and emotional, is still there and this exercise in creative imagination is futile. Thank your mind for its opinion and continue this exercise anyway.

Now replay the same looping image and see yourself, everybody and everything associated with it *unconditionally. Be grateful* for all life experiences, neither good nor bad but simply as opportunities for growth. Overlay *being in-harmony, in-balance, content, fulfilled and in joy*.

The overlays have no specificity. They are not conditional. They are not linked, dependent or attached to any specific person, place or thing.

One way to frame this is to allow or surrender to *thy will be done*, the divine will, rather than individual mind, ego driven self-will. As you engage this exercise, when you think you have released all the images with negative charges and judgments associated with them, now replay the loop again. This time, specifically link the loop of your life story with each parent, sibling, friend, relative, co-worker or boss.

Now add any other person, place, thing or situation and observe whether you are holding an *unconditional,* detached space or not. If not, then the image is not released and we remain bound as effect. Engage the freeze frame, looping, hook removal and overlay *process* in each situation.

When you think or perceive that you have permanently entered the rarified, *unconditional* state of release definitively, then replay your life again and identify any current or chronic symptoms; physical, emotional or mental, any dis-ease states, strong feelings about anything, strong opinions about anything, strong dislikes or likes about anything. Observe whether you are holding an *unconditional*, detached space or not.

Engage the freeze frame, looping, hook removal and overlay *process* as needed.

These symptoms, feelings and opinions represent induction vectors that manifest as body zones of *fascial* twisting, becoming *engrams*. Make this *process* a gift to yourself and your *awakening, healing journey*. Make it a pleasure, joy and challenge, not a burden.

8) Find or start a *Drum Circle* in your area. These are fabulous. This is an expanding world-wide movement to bring us back into alignment with ourselves, each other and Mother Earth.

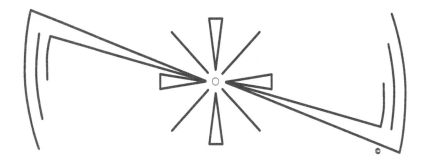

HEALING VIBRATION

Poem by Brett Reeves (*RST patient*)

My morning meditation, a gentle stirring deep within now moistening my eyes.

These words tickled my tongue and beckoned a pen, as the sun began to rise.

Almighty one, pour me, a healing dose so my thirsty cup overflows.

And guide the excess so we may help mend, some other struggling *souls*.

Shadows of trauma always sneaking up from behind to strangle and suffocate.

Blocking meridians, disturbing doshas and choking off *Chi*, closing the essential life force gate.

The voice of truth and freedom is *toning* for me, and *toning* for you.

Simple sounds calling out to a complex pot, of this *hu*man stew.

Inviting the door to open inwardly, illuminating clear steps for our way.

Let the thoughtful silence of wisdom and discernment prevail on our path today.

Unwind this tangled fascial mess, smooth out all the adhered layers that twist and distort.

For my scarred battleship seeks repair in the safe refuge, of a calm and friendly port.

As the solar rays once again gradually dissolve the darkness of the night.

May these glasses of anger, fear and resentment be cleansed, giving way to unobstructed sight.

Might these frequencies, re-tracings and gyrations be the passage way to a new birth.

Plant my feet in a beautiful fragrant garden, firmly *grounding* me, to this amazing mother Earth.

Oh lover of our *soul*, may the path of spiritual awakening be wide enough for more than just a few.

Let ALL feel Thy tug, eager for a healing vibration.

For all things are possible, through you (*HU).*

From my heart,

to your heart.

In Joy,

Lance

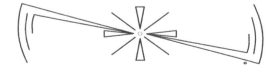

Table of Figures

Fig. 1: **Book Cover: The Edge and Beyond**; Made by Maureen Morris. Background image: Cygnus Loop Supernova Blast, NASA;: NASA copyright policy states that "NASA material is not protected by copyright unless noted". (NASA copyright page or JPL Image) Public Domain

Fig. 2:pg.**48, Gray's Anatomy** 20th ed. 1918, **fig. 503,** Public Domain

Fig. 3: **pg.49, Gray's Anatomy** 20th ed. 1918, **Foot fig. 441**, Public Domain

Fig. 4:**pg.50**, this is a file from the Wikimedia Commons. *It is from the 20th U.S. edition of* **Gray's Anatomy** *of the Human Body,* ***fig#1196, five layers of human scalp*** *originally published in 1918 and therefore lapsed into the public domain.*

Fig. 5:**pg.52**, Dreamstime.com: Royalty free **purchased image stock # 6306392**. This staircase is similar to MC Escher's famous and well recognized painting titled 'Relativity'. The image is to demonstrate graphically the educational principles expressed in this chapter relative to a perception of multiple dimensions in relation to 'String Theory'.

Fig. 6:**pg.53**, this is a file from the Wikimedia Commons. Description= {{Gray's **Anatomy plate Fig.9. |First stages of segmentation of a mammalian ovum.** Semi diagrammatic. (From a drawing by Allen Thomson.) z.p. Zona striata. p.gl. Polar bodies. a. Two-cell stage. b. Four-cell stage. c. Eight-cell stage.). Public Domain.

Fig. 7:**pg.57, Hubble data: NASA**, ESA, and A. Zezas (Harvard-Smithsonian Center for Astrophysics); GALEX data: NASA, JPL-Caltech, GALEX Team, J Huchra et al. (Harvard-Smithsonian Center for Astrophysics); Spitzer data: NASA/JPL/Caltech/S. Willner (Harvard-Smithsonian Center for Astrophysics. This file is in the public domain because it was created by NASA. NASA copyright policy states that "NASA material is not protected by copyright unless noted". (NASA copyright policy page or JPL Image Use Policy)

Fig. 8:**pg.58, North polar hexagonal, cymatic, cloud feature on Saturn,** discovered by Voyager 1 and confirmed in 2006 by Cassini   Credit: NASA/JPL/University of Arizona", Peter Ellis 01:05, 28 March 2007 (UTC)en: Category: Saturn, Source: Originally from en. wikipedia; description page is/was here. Date: 2007-03-28 (first version); 2007-03-28 (last version), Author: Original up loader was Peter Ellis at en. wikipedia Later versions were uploaded by Chris Capoccia at en. wikipedia. Permission: PD-LAYOUT; PD-USGOV-NASA. *This file is in the **public domain** because it was created by NASA.*

Fig. 9:**pg.59***, Original photograph; Blueberry.* Lance Morris

Fig. 10:**pg.59, Original photograph; Bell pepper,** Lance Morris

Fig.11:**pg.65, Description:** A julia set with seed coordinates (-0.156844471694257101941, -0.649707745759247905171).**Source:** English Wikipedia, original upload 25 November 2004 by Eequor. *This image has been released into the **public domain** by its author, Eequor. This applies worldwide.*

Fig. 12:pg.**67**, , MANDELBROT SET; This image is a part of a *set.* The main image in the set is **Mandel zoom 00 mandelbrot set.jpg**. *Permission is granted to copy, distribute and/or modify this document under the terms of the GNU Free Documentation License,*

Fig. 13-26:**pg.68, MULTIPLE PROGRESSIVE FRACTAL IMAGES.** This is a file from the Wikimedia Commons: Created by Wolfgang Beyer with the program *Ultra Fractal 3.* All images of the zoom sequence: 15 pictures. *I, the copyright holder of this work, hereby publish it under the following licenses: Permission is granted to copy, distribute and/or modify this document under the terms of the GNU Free Documentation License,*

Fig. 27:**pg.82, ROMANESCO BROCCOLI (**showing fractal in nature). This is a file from the Wikimedia Commons. Description: Close-up of a remarkable cauliflower showing its fractal properties. We later ate it - it was delicious! Source: Own work (photograph) by up loader. Date: August 24, 2008. Author: AVM Permission: *This file is licensed under the Creative Commons Attribution Share Alike 3.0 License*

Fig. 28:**pg.83, SUTURES (FROM DEER SKULL) AS FRACTALS.** Sutures in a deer skull, 9 February 2008, Author: The green j, Permission *is granted to copy, distribute and/or modify this document under the terms of the GNU Free Documentation License*

Fig. 29: **pg.86, INFANT SKULL, OPEN SUTURES (FONTANEL)** Wikipedia commons: Gray's Anatomy 20th ed. 1918. Fig.197 & 198

Fig. 30:**pg.87, ADULT SKULL CLOSED SUTURES.** Wikipedia Commons: Gray's Anatomy 20th ed. 1918. Fig.188 and 190. Public Domain.

Fig. 31:**pg.101, Gray's Anatomy 20th ed. 1918, fig. 530**, Public Domain

Fig. 32:**pg.106,** This is a file from the Wikimedia Commons. Description; personal drawing. Source; Y Landman. Author; Y Landman. Permission; everyone .*I, the copyright holder of this work, hereby release it into the public domain*

Fig. 33: **pg.113, Gray's Anatomy 20th ed. 1918, hand fig. 425**, Public Domain.

Fig. 34:**pg.117,** A file from the Wikimedia Commons. Description: Archimedean spiral. svg Three 360° turnings of one arm of an Archimedean spiral. Source: Own work; based on Image: Archimedean spiral.png by User: Anon Moos. Date 7 June 2006,(2006-06-07) Author Shaun A. Hill, Permission (Reusing this image) CC-BY-SA-2.*This file is licensed under the Creative Commons Attribution Share Alike 2.5 License. In short: you are free to share and make derivative works of the file under the conditions that you appropriately attribute it, and that you distribute it only under a license identical to this one.*

Fig. 35:**pg.117, Spiral/ Helix/ conical Helix:** *Made by J. Randall Harris under contract from Dr. Morris for this manuscript.*

Fig. 36: **pg.122, Yin/ Yang symbol**, Date 7 December 2007,(2007-12-07) Author : Klem *I, the copyright holder of this work,* hereby publish it under the following licenses: from Wikipedia, Permission is granted to copy, distribute and/or modify this document under the terms of the GNU Free Documentation License, Version 1.2 or any later version.

Fig. 37:**pg.145, Original Photograph by Maureen Morris.** Used with permission.

Fig. 38:**pg.155, DNA HELIX NEBULAE** (Public Domain; courtesy of NASA)

Fig. 39:**pg.155,** This is a file from the Wikimedia Commons. Description; The golden ratio (phi) represented as a line divided into two segments a and b, such that the entire line is to the longer a segment as the a segment is to the shorter b segment. Source; en: Image: Golden ratio line.png. Date; 23 March 2007. Author; Traced by User: Stannered. Permission; *This image is **ineligible for** copyright and therefore in the **public domain***

Fig. 40:**pg.157,** This is a file from the Wikimedia Commons. Description; Uppercase and lowercase Greek letter phi, the 21th letter of the Greek alphabet. Times New Roman font. Source; Own work. Date; 3 January 2006. Author; Dcoetzee, F l a n k e r Permission; *This image is **ineligible for** copyright and therefore in the public domain*

Fig. 41:**pg.158, DNA** This is a file from the Wikimedia Commons: An overview of the structure of DNA. Created by Michael Ströck (mstroeck) on February 8, 2006. Released under the GFDL. Permission is granted to copy, distribute and/or modify this document under the terms of the **GNU Free Documentation License**

Fig. 42:**pg.159,** This is a file from the Wikimedia Commons. Description; **Fibonacci spiral** with square sizes up to 34. Source; self-drawn in Inkscape. Date; 17 March 2008. Author; This media is lacking **author** information. Permission; *I, the copyright holder of this work, hereby release it into the **public domain.***

Fig. 43:**pg.190,** Dreamstime.com: Royalty free **purchased image stock # 6279077. Concentric rings in water.**

Fig. 44:**pg.191,** Dreamstime.com: Royalty free **purchased image stock # 3215939. Criss-crossing interference patterns in water.**

Fig. 45:**pg.203,** Original jpeg by Michael Kelley, permission from creator.

Fig. 46:**pg.236, Sphere** Made under contract to Dr. Morris by J. Randall Harris

Fig. 47:**pg. 238,**This is a file from the Wikimedia Commons. Description; **Dispersion of light inside a prism.** Now with waves. Source; Self. Date; 24 December 2007. Author; Lucas V. Barbosa. Permission; Public Domain

Fig. 48.**pg. 330, Original diagram by;** Lance Morris

Fig. 49:**pg.335,** Foot Reflexology Chart; permission from Littleepiphany.com

REFERENCE & BIBLIOGRAPHY NOTES

A majority of my reference and bibliography notes are from an Internet resource named Wikipedia; *a multilingual, web-based, free-content encylopedia project supported by the Wikimedia Foundation and based on an openly editable model.* I have done this intentionally. If you have purchased a copy of my book as an E-book you can immediately use all the blue highlighted and underlined hyper-links. This offers a wonderful opportunity to expand your information base about any author or topic in my book.

If your book is a hard copy, you can follow and access all the same links by going to www.wikipedia.org through your computer. Wikipedia offers an astute collection of thumbnail descriptions, images, and encyclopedia articles about a wide spectrum of topic-categories. I highly recommend supporting and using them. I dedicate a special thank you to Wikipedia. As well as the common way of listing an individual reference or bibligraphy source, I often give you a Wikipedia referenced specific source with a part of their thumbnail article attached, plus all their expanded links. This is a fabulous resource. Please use this bibliography liberally. It's extremely entertaining and informative in its own right and the links make it a great tool.

In technical or scientific circles, Wikipedia is often construed as an inadequate reference source. This is an unfair characterization, as Wikipedia does not restrict or limit original references, but verifies, expands and adds to them using only reliable published sources.

1. **pg. 44,** From Wikipedia: The **Big Bang** is the cosmological model of the initial conditions and subsequent development of the Universe that is supported by the most comprehensive and accurate explanations from current scientific and observation.[1][2] As used by cosmologists, the term *Big Bang* generally refers to the idea that the Universe has expanded from a primordial hot and dense initial condition at some finite time in the past (currently estimated to have been approximately 13.7 billion years ago[3]), and continues to expand to this day.

2. **pg. 44,** From Wikipedia: n physics, a **unified field theory** is a type of field theory that allows all of the fundamental between elementary particles to be written in terms of a single field. There is no accepted unified field theory yet, and this remains an open line of research. The term was coined by Albert Einstein who attempted to unify the general theory of relativity with electromagnetism. A Theory of Everything is closely related to unified field theory, but differs by not requiring the basis of nature to be fields, and also attempts to explain all physical constants of nature. According to the current understanding of physics, forces between objects (e.g. gravitation) are not transmitted directly between the two objects, but instead go through intermediary entities called fields. All four of the known fundamental forces are mediated by fields, which in the Standard Model of particle physics result from exchange of bosons (integral-spin particles). Specifically the four interactions to be unified are (from strongest to weakest):

- Strong nuclear: the interaction responsible for holding quarks together to form neutrons and protons, and holding neutrons and protons together to form nuclei. The exchange particle that mediates this force is the gluon.
- Electromagnetic interaction: the familiar interaction that acts on electrically charged particles. The photon is the exchange particle for this force.
- Weak nuclear: a repulsive short-range interaction responsible for some forms of radioactivity, that acts on electrons, neutrinos, and quarks. It is governed by the W and Z bosons.
- Gravitational interaction: a long-range attractive interaction that acts on *all* particles with mass. The postulated exchange particle has been named the graviton.

Modern unified field theory attempts to bring these four force-mediating fields together into a single framework. Quantum theory seems to limit any deterministic theory's descriptive power (in simple terms, no theory can predict events more accurately than allowed by the Planck constant).

3. **pg. 47,** From Wikipedia: **Déjà vu** «already seen»; also called paramnesia, from Greek παρα "para," "near, against, contrary to" + μνήμη "mnēmē," "memory») or **promnesia**, is the experience of feeling sure that one has witnessed or experienced a new situation previously (an individual feels as though an event has already happened or has happened in the recent past), although the exact circumstances of the previous encounter are uncertain. The term was coined by a French psychic researcher, Émile Boirac (1851–1917) in his book *L'Avenir des sciences psychiques* ("The Future of Psychic Sciences"), which expanded upon an essay he wrote while an undergraduate. The experience of déjà vu is usually accompanied by a compelling sense of familiarity, and also a sense of "eeriness", "strangeness", or "weirdness". The "previous" experience is most frequently attributed to a dream, although in some cases there is a firm sense that the experience "genuinely happened" in the past.[1]

4.   pg. 50, Lipton, B.H. *The Biology of Belief*: *Unleashing the power of consciousness, Matter and Miracles*. Santa Rosa: Elite books, 2005. From Wikipedia: Dr. **Bruce Lipton** is an American geneticist, who attempts to "bridge the gap that was formed some 150 - 200 years ago, when the French biologist Jean-Baptiste de Lamarck and later Charles Darwin published, amongst other writings Species". Lipton promotes the idea that genes and DNA can be manipulated by our beliefs [1]. Biography: **Bruce H. Lipton** is a former research scientist from Stanford University School of Medicine. His main area of research is that of bridging science and spirit. He has been a guest speaker on television and radio shows, as well as a keynote presenter for national conferences.

5.   pg. 51, From Wikipedia: **String theory** posits that the electrons and quarks within an atom are not 0-dimensional objects, but 1-dimensional strings. These strings can move and vibrate, giving the observed particles their flavor, charge, mass and spin. The strings make closed loops unless they encounter surfaces, called D-branes, where they can open up into 1-dimensional lines. The endpoints of the string cannot break off the D-brane, but they can slide around on it. String theory is a theory of gravity, an extension of General Relativity, and the classical interpretation of strings and branes is that they are quantum vibrating, extended charged black holes. The overarching physical insight behind string theory is the holographic principle, which states that the description of the oscillations of the surface of a black hole must also describe the space-time around it. Holography demands that a low-dimensional theory describing the fluctuations of a horizon will end up describing everything that can fall through, which can be anything at all. So a theory of a black hole horizon is a theory of everything.

6.   pg. 51, From Wikipedia: On **M-Theory**; String theory then ran into a problem: another version of the equations was discovered; then another, and then another. Eventually, there were five major string theories, all based on a 10-dimensional universe, and all of them appeared to be correct. Scientists were not comfortable with five seemingly contradictory sets of equations to describe the same thing. In the mid 90s, a string theorist named Edward Witten of the Institute for Advanced Study and other important researchers considered that the five different versions of string theory might be describing the same thing seen from different perspectives. They proposed a unifying theory called "M-Theory", in which the "M" is not specifically defined, but is generally understood to stand for "membrane." M-Theory brought all of the string theories together. It did this by asserting that strings are really 1-dimensional slices of a 2-dimensional membrane vibrating in 11-dimensional space.

7.   pg. 55, From Wikipedia: **Hatha Yoga** (Sanskrit *haṭha yoga,* IPA: also called Hatha Vidya , is a system of Yoga introduced by Yogi Swatmarama, a sage of 15th century India, and compiler of the Hatha Yoga Pradipika. In this treatise Swatmarama introduces Hatha Yoga as preparatory stage of physical purification that the body practices for higher meditation. The Asanas and Pranayama in Raja Yoga were what the Hindu Yogis used to physically train their body for long periods of meditation. This practice is called *shatkarma*. The word Hatha is a compound of the words *Ha* and *Tha* meaning sun and moon , referring to Praana and Apaana, and also to the principle nadis (energy channels) of the subtle body that must be fully operational to attain a state of dhyana or samādhi. According to the Moneir-Williams Sanskrit Dictionary, the word "hatha" means forceful. It is a strong practice done for purification.

348

In other respects Hatha yoga follows the same principles as the Raaja Yoga of Patanjali including moral restraint *yama* and spiritual observances *niyama*. Hatha Yoga is what most people in the West associate with the word "Yoga" and is practiced for mental and physical health throughout the West.

8. pg. 55, From Wikipedia: **Surat Shabd Yoga** or **Surat Shabda Yoga** is a form of spiritual practice that is followed in the Sant Mat and many other related spiritual traditions. As a Sanskrit term, *Surat* means "soul," *shabd* means "word" and *yoga* means "union." The term "word" means the "Sound Current," the "Audible Life Stream" or the "Essence of the Absolute Supreme Being," that is, the dynamic force of creative energy that was sent out, as sound vibration, from the Supreme Being into the abyss of space at the dawn of the universe's manifestation, and that is being sent forth, through the ages, framing all things that constitute and inhabit the universe.[1].The etymology of "Surat Shabda Yoga" presents its purpose: the "Union of the Soul with the Essence of the Absolute Supreme Being." Other expressions for Surat Shabda Yoga include Sehaj Yoga (an easy path leading to Sehaj or equipoise) The Path of Light and Sound, The Path of the Sants, The Journey of Soul, and The Yoga of the Sound Current.

9. pg. 56, John 1:1, Bible; King James Version

10. pg. 57, From Wikipedia: **Cymatics** (from Greek: κῦμα «wave»), also known as **modal phenomena**, is the study of visible sound and vibration, typically on the surface of a plate, diaphragm, or membrane. Directly visualizing vibrations involves using sound to excite media often in the form of particles, pastes, and liquids. [1].The apparatus employed can be simple, such as a Chladni Plate [2] or advanced such as the Cyma Scope, a laboratory instrument that makes visible the inherent geometries within sound and music.

11. pg. 57, Braden, Gregg 'Awakening to Zero Point: The Collective Initiation' Video set: Bellevue WA, Radio Bookstore Press. 1996

12. pg. 58, From Wikipedia: **Hans Jenny** (1904-1972) was a physician and natural scientist who is considered the father of cymatics, the study of wave phenomena. Jenny was born in Basel, Switzerland. After completing his doctorate, he taught science at the Rudolph Steiner School in Zürich for four years before beginning his medical practice. In 1967, Jenny published the first volume of *Cymatics: The Study of Wave Phenomena.* The second volume came out in 1972, the year he died.

This book was a written and photographic documentation of the effects of sound vibrations on fluids, powders, and liquid paste. He concluded, "This is not an unregulated chaos; it is a dynamic but ordered pattern." Jenny made use of crystal oscillators and an invention of his own by the name of the tonoscope to set plates and membranes vibrating. With the tonoscope, quartz sand is spread onto a black drum membrane which is 60cm in diameter. The membrane is set into vibrations by singing rather loudly through a cardboard pipe. The sand now produces complex symmetrical forms, known as Chladni patterns named after Ernst Chladni who discovered this phenomenon in 1787. Low tones result in rather simple and clear pictures, while higher tones form more complex structures.[1]

13. pg. 60, From Wikipedia: *Powers of Ten* is a 1977 short documentary film written and directed by Ray Eames and her husband, Charles Eames.[1] The film depicts the relative scale of the Universe in factors of ten (see also logarithmic scale and order of magnitude). The film is an adaptation of the 1957 book *Cosmic View* by Kees Boeke, and more recently is the basis of a new book version. Both adaptations, film and book, follow the form of the Boeke original, adding color and photography to the black and white drawings employed by Boeke in his seminal work. In 1998, "Powers of Ten" was selected for preservation in the United States National Film Registry by the Library of Congress as being "culturally, historically, or aesthetically significant". The film begins with an overhead image of a man and woman reclining on a blanket; the view is that of one meter across. The viewpoint, accompanied by expository voiceover by Philip Morrison, then slowly zooms out to a view ten meters across (or 10^1 m in standard form), revealing that the man is picnicking in a park with a female companion. The zoom-out continues (at a rate of one power of ten per 10 seconds), to a view of 100 meters (10^2 m), then 1 kilometer (10^3 m), and so on, increasing the perspective—the picnic is revealed to be taking place in Burnham Park, near Soldier Field on Chicago's lakefront—and continuing to zoom out to a field of view of 10^{24} meters, or the size of the observable universe. The camera then zooms back in at a rate of a power of ten per 2 seconds to the picnic, and then slows back down to its original rate into the man's hand, to views of negative powers of ten—10^{-1} m (10 centimeters), and so forth—until the camera comes to quarks in a proton of a carbon atom at 10^{-16} meter.

14. pg. 63, From Wikipedia: **William James** (January 11, 1842 – August 26, 1910) was a pioneering American psychologist and philosopher trained as a medical doctor. He wrote influential books on the young science of psychology, educational psychology, psychology of religious experience and mysticism, and the philosophy of pragmatism.

15. pg. 63, From Wikipedia: **Rudolf Otto** (September 25, 1869–6 March1937) was an eminent German Lutheran theologian and scholar of comparative religion. **Numinous** (pronounced /nuːmɪnəs, njuːmɪnəs/) (from the Classical Latin *numen*) is an English adjective describing the power or presence of a divinity. The word was popularized in the early twentieth century by the German theologian Rudolf Otto in his influential book *Das Heilige* (1917; translated into English as *The Idea of the Holy*, 1923). According to Otto the numinous experience has two aspects: *mysterium tremendum*, which is the tendency to invoke fear and trembling; and *mysterium fascinans*, the tendency to attract, fascinate and compel.The numinous experience also has a personal quality to it, in that the person feels to be in communion with a *wholly other*. The numinous experience can lead in different cases to belief in deities, the supernatural, the sacred, the holy, and the transcendent.

16. pg. 64, Heinlein, Robert 'Stranger in a Strange Land', New York, Penguin Publishing, 1961

17. pg. 65, From Wikipedia: **Benoît B. Mandelbrot** [1] (born 20 November 1924) is a French American mathematician, best known as the father of fractal geometry. He is Sterling Professor of Mathematical Sciences, Emeritus at Yale University; IBM Fellow Emeritus at the Thomas J. Watson Research Center; and Battelle Fellow at the Pacific Northwest National Laboratory. He was born in Poland. His family moved to France when he was a child, and he was educated in France. He is a dual French and American citizen. Mandelbrot now lives and works in the United States.

18. pg. 98, From Institute of **HeartMath** web-site: IHM is a recognized, global leader in emotional physiology, stress management and the physiology of heart-brain research. The HeartMath Research Center is engaged in basic psychophysiology, neurocardiology and biophysics research, and in clinical, workplace and organizational intervention and treatment outcome studies in collaboration with numerous university and health care system partners. Our research has significantly advanced the understanding of heart-brain interactions, heart-rhythm-pattern and heart-rate-variability analyses, emotional physiology and the physiology of optimal learning and performance. Expanding areas interest at the Institute of HeartMath include furthering scientific understanding of the human biofield, intuition and the emotional energetic system. The Global Coherence Monitoring System a forefront project that will examine the energetic resonance between the earth's magnetic field and the rhythms of human heart and brain activity. Other expanding areas of interest at the HeartMath Research Center include furthering scientific understanding of the human biofield, intuition and the emotional energetic system.

19. pg. 114, From Wikipedia: **Kundalini yoga** is a physical and meditative discipline within the tradition of Yoga, associated with the subdivision of hatha yoga [1]. It describes a set of advanced yoga exercises. The exercises are also sometimes referred to as Kriya Yoga or simply Kriya. According to Hindu tradition Kundalini yoga is a pure spiritual science that leads to enlightenment and God-Realization under the guidance of a Spiritual Master. The awakening of kundalini means awakening of inner knowledge [2]. According to Hindu philosophy Kundalini is a concentrated form of prana or life force, lying dormant in chakras in the body. It is conceptualized as a coiled up serpent (literally, 'kundalini' in Sanskrit is 'That which is coiled.' Sanskrit kund, "to burn"; kunda, "to coil or to spiral"). The serpent is considered to be female, coiled up three and a half times, with its mouth engulfing the base of the Sushumna nadi. In the classical literature of Kashmir Shaivism kundalini is described in three different manifestations.

The first of these is as the universal energy or para-kundalini. The second of these is as the energizing function of the body-mind complex or prana-kundalini. The third of these is as consciousness or shakti-kundalini which simultaneously subsumes and intermediates between these two. Ultimately these three forms are the same but understanding these three different forms will help to understand the different manifestations of kundalini.[3] The path of Kundalini is said to proceed from the Muladhara Chakra at the lower end of the spinal column up to the Sahasara Chakra at the top of the head. But its awakening is not thought to be a physical occurrence; it consists exclusively of a development in consciousness. According to some sources, awakening of kundalini brings with it pure joy, pure knowledge and pure love [2]. According to one source, those people who write about supposed danger of this path either do not have a (self-realized) master or do not follow his instructions.[2] According to one source, the word kundalini literally means "the curl of the lock of hair of the beloved." [4][5]. It is a metaphor, a poetic way of describing the flow of energy and consciousness which already is said to exist within each person. The practices are said to enable the person to merge with or "yoke" the universal Self.

This merging of individual consciousness with the universal consciousness is said to create a "divine union" called "yoga"[6]. Kundalini yoga is sometimes called "the yoga of awareness" because it awakens the "kundalini" which is the unlimited potential that already exists within every human being[7]

20. **pg. 116,** From Wikipedia: **Albert Einstein** 14 March 1879–18 April 1955) was a theoretical physicist. His many contributions to physics include the special and general theories of relativity, the founding of relativistic, the first post-Newtonian expansion, explaining the perihelion advance of Mercury, prediction of the deflection of light and gravitational lensing, the first fluctuation dissipation theorem which explained the Brownian movement, the photon theory and wave-particle duality, the quantum, the zero-point energy concept, the semi classical version of the Schrödinger equation, and the quantum theory of a monatomic gas which predicted Bose-Einstein condensation. Einstein is best known for his theories of special relativity and general relativity. He received the 1921 Nobel Prize in Physics "for his services to Theoretical Physics, and especially for his discovery of the law of the photoelectric effect."[2] Einstein published more than and over 150 non-scientific works.[3] He is often regarded as the father of modern physics. [4]Special relativity Main article: History of special relativity His 1905 paper on the electrodynamics of moving bodies introduced his theory of special relativity, which showed that the observed independence of the speed of light on the observer's state of motion required fundamental changes to the notion of simultaneity. Consequences of this include the time of a moving body slowing down and contracting (in the direction of motion) relative to the frame of the observer. This paper also argued that the idea of a luminiferous aether – one of the leading theoretical entities in physics at the time – was superfluous.[34] In his paper on mass–energy equivalence, which had previously considered to be distinct concepts, Einstein deduced from his equations of special relativity what has been called the twentieth century's best-known equation: $E = mc^2$.[35][36] This equation suggests that tiny amounts of mass could be converted into huge amounts of energy and presaged the development of nuclear.[37]

Einstein's 1905 work on relativity remained controversial for many years, but was accepted by leading physicists, starting with Max Planck.[38] [39. General Relativity: This theory explains gravitation as distortion of the structure of space-time by matter, affecting the inertial motion of other matter.

21. **pg. 117,** From Wikipedia: **Archimedes of Syracuse** (Greek: Άρχιμήδης; c. 287 BC – c. 212 BC) was a Greek mathematician, physicist, engineer, inventor, and astronomer. Although few details of his life are known, he is regarded as one of the leading scientists in classical antiquity. Among his advances in physics are the foundations of hydrostatics, statics and the explanation of the principle of the lever. He is credited with designing innovative machines, including siege engines and the screw pump that bears his name. Archimedes is generally considered to be the greatest mathematician of antiquity and one of the greatest of all time.[2] [3] He used the method of exhaustion to calculate the area under the arc of a parabola with the summation of an infinite series, and gave a remarkably accurate approximation of pi.[4] He also defined the spiral bearing his name, formulas for the volumes of surfaces of revolution and an ingenious system for expressing very large numbers.

22. **pg. 118,** From Wikipedia: *Qigong* (or *ch'i kung*) is an internal Chinese meditative practice which often uses slow graceful movements and controlled breathing techniques to promote the circulation of qi within the human body, and enhance a practitioner's overall health. There are also many forms of Qigong that are done with little or no movement at all, in standing, sitting and supine positions; likewise, not all forms of Qigong use breath control techniques.

Although not a martial art, qigong is often confused with the Chinese martial art of tai chi. This misunderstanding can be attributed to the fact that most Chinese martial arts practitioners will usually also practice some form of qigong and to the uninitiated, these arts may seem to be alike. There are more than 10,000 styles of qigong and 200 million people practicing these methods. There are three main reasons why people do qigong: 1) To gain strength, improve health or reverse a disease 2) To gain skill working with qi, so as to become a healer 3) To become more connected with the "Tao, God, True Source, Great Spirit", for a more meaningful connection with nature and the universe. In its simplest form, the Chinese character for qi, in qigong, can mean air, breath, or "life force". Gong means work, so qigong is therefore the practice of "working" with ones "life force". The term was not widely known until the 1970s during a period some call the "Qigong Wave" where groups of 10,000-40,000 people regularly gathered inside Chinese stadiums to practice qigong together. Some in the Chinese government became concerned that one quasi-religious/political group (see Falun Dafa or Falun Gong) who practiced a Qigong form of their own, might turn into a political weapon, and in 1999, banned all large qigong gatherings. Currently there is a movement underway in China, the United States, and Europe to preserve the valuable aspects of these traditional Chinese practices and to have them studied using Western scientific methods. Attitudes toward a scientific basis for qigong vary markedly.

Most Western medical practitioners and many practitioners of traditional Chinese medicine, as well as the Chinese government, view qigong as a set of breathing and movement exercises, with possible benefits to health through stress reduction and exercise. Other practitioners view qigong in more metaphysical terms, claiming that qi can be felt as a vibration or electrical current and physically circulated through channels called meridians. Many testify to a reduction or elimination of pain through the use of qigong.

23. **pg. 118,** From Wikipedia: **Tai chi chuan** (simplified Chinese: 太极拳; traditional Chinese: 太極拳; pinyin: tàijíquán; Wade–Giles: t'ai¹ chi² ch'üan²) is an internal Chinese martial art often practiced for health reasons. Tai chi is typically practiced for a variety of other personal reasons: its hard and soft martial art technique, demonstration competitions, health and longevity. Consequently, a multitude of training forms exist, both traditional and modern, which correspond to those aims. Some of tai chi chuan's training forms are well known to Westerners as the slow motion routines that groups of people practice together every morning in parks around the world, particularly in China. Today, tai chi has spread worldwide. Most modern styles of tai chi trace their development to at least one of the five traditional schools: Chen, Yang, Wu/Hao, Wu and Sun.

24. **pg. 118,** From Wikipedia; **Sufism** (Arabic: تَصَوُّف taṣawwuf,(Persian: تصوّف گری) also spelled as tasavvuf and tasavvof according to the Persian pronunciation, is generally understood to be the inner, mystical dimension of Islam. [1][2][3]

A practitioner of this tradition is generally known as a ṣūfī (صُوفِيّ), though some adherents of the tradition reserve this term only for those practitioners who have attained the goals of the Sufi tradition. Another name used for the Sufi seeker is dervish. Classical Sufi scholars have defined Sufism as "a science whose objective is the reparation of the heart and turning it away from all else but God."[4]

Alternatively, in the words of the renowned Darqawi Sufi teacher Ahmad ibn Ajiba, "a science through which one can know how to travel into the presence of the Divine, purify one's inner self from filth, and beautify it with a variety of praiseworthy traits."[5]**Islam** (Arabic: الإسلام‎ *al-'islām,* pronounced [ʔislæːm] (🔊listen)[note 1]) is the religion articulated by the Qur'an, a book considered by its adherents to be the verbatim word of the single incomparable God (Arabic: الله‎ Allāh), and by the Islamic prophet Muhammad's demonstrations and real-life examples (called the Sunnah, collected through narration of his companions in collections of Hadith). The word *Islam* is a homograph, having multiple meanings, and a triliteral of the word salaam, which directly translates as *peace.* Other meanings include submission, or the total surrender of oneself to God (see Islam (term)).[1] When the two root words are put together, the word 'Islam' gives the meaning 'Peace acquired by submission to the will of God'. An adherent of Islam is a Muslim, meaning "one who submits (to God)".[2],[3] The word *Muslim* is the active participle of the same verb of which *Islām* is the infinitive. Muslims regard their religion as the completed and universal version of a monotheistic faith revealed at many times and places before, including, notably, to the prophets Abraham, Moses and Jesus. Islamic tradition holds that previous messages and revelations have been changed and distorted over time

The **Mawlawi Order**, or the **Mevlevilik** or **Mevleviye** (Persian: مولویه - *Mowlawīya*) are a Sufi order founded in Konya (in present-day Turkey) by the followers of Jalal ad-Din Muhammad Balkhi-Rumi, a 13th century Persian poet, Islamic jurist, and theologian. They are also known as the **Whirling Dervishes** due to their famous practice of whirling as a form of dhikr (remembrance of God). Dervish is a common term for an initiate of the Sufi path; the whirling is part of the formal Sema ceremony and the participants are properly known as semazens.[1

25.   pg. 118, Bio Energetic Synchronization Technique (B.E.S.T.) Developed during the mid-1970s by chiropractor **Milton Ted Morter, Jr.,** of Rogers, Arkansas, is claimed to be "a holistic program that coordinates and balances the workings of all the systems of the body." [1] Morter defines B.E. S.T. as "a nonforceful chiropractic technique for the 21st century that removed interference from the nervous system by the use of the hands." [2] Morter claims that such interferences occur when "subtle pulses" in different parts of the body are not "synchronized." [3] From www.chirobase.org homepage. B.E.S.T. is a non-forceful, energy balancing hands on procedure used to help reestablish the full healing potential of the body. Understanding the body makes no mistakes regarding health and longevity, B.E.S.T. principles acknowledge the concept of Interference we create with our conscious mind. This Interference caused imbalance in the autonomic nervous system leading to exhaustion of our organ systems over time. Researched at major universities, taught in several Chiropractic Colleges and in professional continuing education seminars, B.E.S.T. is recognized as an effective healing science. The principles and concepts of Morter Health System and B.E.S.T. technique are available to families, therapists and health care practitioners, from www.morter.com homepage.

26.   pg. 118, From Wikipedia: **Craniosacral therapy** (also called **CST, cranial osteopathy,** also spelled **CranioSacral** bodywork or therapy) is an alternative medicine therapy used by osteopaths, massage, naturopaths, chiropractors, physical, and occupational therapists. A craniosacral therapy session involves the therapist placing their hands on the patient, which they say allows them to tune into what they call the craniosacral system.[1] The practitioner gently works with the spine and the skull and its cranial sutures, diaphragms, and fascia.

In this way, the restrictions of nerve passages are said to be eased, the movement of cerebrospinal fluid through the spinal cord is said to be optimized, and misaligned bones are said to be restored to their proper position. Craniosacral therapists use the therapy to treat mental stress, neck and back pain, migraines, TMJ Syndrome, and for chronic pain conditions such as fibromyalgia.[2][3][4] Several studies have reported that there is little scientific support for major elements of the underlying theoretical model, which has not been rigorously analyzed.[5] History: Cranial Osteopathy was originated by physician William Sutherland, DO (1873-1954) in 1898-1900. While looking at a disarticulated skull, Sutherland was struck by the idea that the cranial sutures of the temporal where they meet the parietal bones were *"beveled, like the gills of a fish, indicating articular mobility for a respiratory mechanism."*[6] This idea that the bones of the skull could move was contrary to North American contemporary anatomical belief. Sutherland stated the dural membranes act as 'guy-wires' for the movement of the cranial bones, holding tension for the opposite motion. He used the term *reciprocal tension membrane system* (RTM) to describe the three Cartesian axes held in reciprocal tension, or tensegrity, creating the cyclic movement of inhalation and exhalation of the cranium.

The RTM as described by Sutherland includes the spinal dura, with an attachment to the sacrum. After his observation of the cranial mechanism, Sutherland stated that the sacrum moves synchronously with the cranial bones. Sutherland began to teach this work to other osteopaths from about the 1930s, and continued to do so until his death. His work was at first largely rejected by the mainstream osteopathic profession as it challenged some of the closely held beliefs among practitioners of the time. In the 1940s the American School of Osteopathy started a post-graduate course called 'Osteopathy in the Cranial Field' directed by Sutherland, and was followed by other schools. This new branch of practice became known as "cranial osteopathy". As knowledge of this form of treatment began to spread, Sutherland trained more teachers to meet the demand, notably Drs Viola Frymann, Edna Lay, Howard Lippincott, Anne Wales, Chester Handy and Rollin Becker. The Cranial Academy was established in the US in 1947, and continues to teach DOs, MDs, and Dentists "an expansion of the general principles of osteopathy"[7] including a special understanding of the central nervous system and primary respiration. Towards the end of his life Sutherland believed that he began to sense a "power" which generated corrections from inside his clients' bodies without the influence of external forces applied by him as the therapist. Similar to Qi and Prana, this contact with, what he perceived to be the Breath of Life changed his entire treatment focus to one of spiritual reverence and subtle touch.[8] This spiritual approach to the work has come to be known as both 'biodynamic' craniosacral therapy and 'biodynamic' osteopathy, and has had further contributions from practitioners such as Becker and James Jealous (biodynamic osteopathy), and Franklyn Sills (biodynamic craniosacral therapy). The biodynamic approach recognizes that embryological forces direct the embryonic cells to create the shape of the body, and places importance on recognition of these formative patterns for maximum therapeutic benefit, as this enhances the ability of the patient to access their health as an expression of the original intention of their existence. From 1975 to 1983, osteopathic physician John E. Upledger and neurophysiologist and histologist Ernest W. Retzlaff worked at Michigan State University as clinical researchers and professors. They set up a team of anatomists, physiologists, biophysicists, and bioengineers to investigate the pulse he had observed and study further Sutherland's theory of cranial bone movement.

Upledger and Retzlaff went on to publish their results, which they interpreted as support for both the concept of cranial bone movement and the concept of a cranial rhythm.[9][10][11] Later reviews of these studies have concluded that their research is of insufficient quality to provide conclusive proof for the effectiveness of craniosacral therapy and the existence of cranial bone movement.[12]

Upledger developed his own treatment style, and when he started to teach his work to a group of students who were not osteopaths he generated the term 'CranioSacral therapy', based on the corresponding movement between cranium and sacrum. Craniosacral therapists often (although not exclusively) work more directly with the emotional and psychological aspects of the patient than osteopaths working in the cranial field [citation needed]. Craniosacral Therapy Associations have been formed in the UK, [13] North America, [14] and Australia.[15]

27.   **Pg.118,** From Wikipedia: **The Trager Approach** is a mind-body approach to movement education. It is a system of gentle, rhythmic movement and touch aimed at facilitating deep relaxation, increased physical mobility, and promoting the body's optimal performance. There are several aspects of the approach: one in which the client passively receives the movement work on a padded table from a *Trager* practitioner; and another aspect, in which the client is taught to actively explore comfortable, free movement for themselves, is called *Mentastics*. Underlying to the basic aim of psychophysical integration in the *Trager* Approach, is a form of neuromuscular re-education called Reflex Response. This aspect of Dr. Trager's work actively involves the client in awakening the connection between mind and body. **Development:** The *Trager* Approach was the creation of a single individual, Milton Trager, M.D. He first encountered its principles intuitively during physical exercise, at the age of 18. He then spent the next 50 years, first as a lay practitioner and later as a medical professional, expanding and refining his approach. Dr. Trager died in 1997. Dr. Trager's first student, Betty Fuller, became the first teacher of his work and, with Dr. Trager, organized the Trager Institute in 1979. Dr. Milton Trager's work is now carried on by Trager International and the instructors and certified practitioners of the *Trager* Approach.[1]

28.   **pg. 118,** From Wikipedia; The **Feldenkrais** Method was originated by **Dr Moshé Feldenkrais** (1904-1984), a Ukrainian-born Jewish physicist and judo practitioner who moved to Israel and eventually became an Israeli. The **Feldenkrais Method** is an educational system centered on movement, aiming to expand and refine the use of the self through awareness.[1] It is intended for those who wish to improve their movement repertoire (dancers, musicians, artists), as well as those wishing to reduce pain or limitations in movement, and many who want to improve their general well-being and personal development. Because it uses movement as the primary vehicle for gaining awareness, it is directly applicable to disorders that arise from restricted or habitually poor movement. But as a process for gaining awareness, the system claims to expand a person's choices and responses to many aspects of life: emotions, relationships, and intellectual tasks; and it applies at any level, from severe disorder to highly professional performance. The Feldenkrais Method holds that there is no separation between mind and body, and thus learning to move better can improve one's overall well-being on many levels. [citation needed]. The Feldenkrais Method is often regarded as complementary medicine.[2] However, Feldenkrais practitioners generally don't regard their work as "treatment" or "cure," because they are not working from the medical model. Instead of directly working a change to the physical body, they are working with the nervous system and enabling discovery of new choices.[1]

29.   **pg. 118,** From Wikipedia: **Polarity therapy** is a holistic alternative medicine health system developed in the 1940s by Randolph Stone.[1] Proponents claim healing can be achieved through manipulation of what they describe as complementary (or polarized) forces, a form of putative energy.[2] The term Stone borrowed from Chinese philosophy to describe those forces is yin and yang. The practice is unsupported by evidence.[3][1] Polarity therapy is a synthesis of ancient Eastern and alternative medicine health care ideas, centered on the concept of a human.[4]

Using touch, verbal interaction, exercise, nutrition and other methods,[5] practitioners of polarity therapy seek to balance and restore the natural flow of energy which, it is claimed,[who?] flows from the universe and into the body through the chakras. The aim is to re-establish "balance". In addition to polarity bodywork, specific polarity yoga exercises, counseling/positive thinking, and nutritional recommendations are claimed to enhance vitality. Between 1947 and 1954, Stone published seven books describing polarity therapy principles and applications. These were subsequently consolidated into three volumes: **Polarity Therapy** Vol. I and Vol. II (CRCS, 1986), and **Health-Building** (The Book Publishing Co., 1999), **Principles of Polarity Therapy**.[6]Advocates and practitioners of PT claim that a subtle, invisible and intangible energetic system is the substrate for all phenomena. According to proponents, if the energetic flow is corrected and restored to its original design, the form will follow.

Further, they claim that blockages in the flow of energy lead to pain and disease (directly contradicting the germ theory), or be experienced as stuck emotions and lack of vitality. They claim that this is similar to the measurable and quantifiable electromagnetic bond between electron and proton that forms atoms, a claim which is not scientific, but pseudoscience. There is no scientific basis for this belief, nor any reproducible measurements of this system. While an electromagnetic metaphor is often used, Stone emphasized that the energy concept had a larger context; he referred to it as the "Breath of Life"[7] and used esoteric language (such as *ki, ch'i, prana* and *life force*) from spiritual traditions (especially mystic Christianity,[8]Ayurveda,[9]Taoism, Hinduism[10], Buddhism,[11]Sufism and Yoga[12]) to describe PT.

30. pg. 118, From Wikipedia: **Rolfing** is the commonly used name for the system of Structural Integration soft tissue manipulation founded by **Ida Pauline Rolf**[1] in the 1950s. The terms Rolfing and Rolfer are trademarks of The Rolf Institute of Structural Integration.[2]The Rolf Institute of Structural Integration states that Rolfing is a "holistic system of soft tissue manipulation and movement education that organized the whole body in gravity".[3] Claims include that clients stand straighter, gain height, and move better through the correction of soft tissue fixations or improper tonus. A 2004 review of Rolfing found that "there is no evidence-based literature to support Rolfing in any specific disease group".[4]History: Ida Pauline Rolf developed a method in the early to mid 1940s with the goal of organizing the human structure in relation to gravity. This method was originally called *Postural Release* and later *Structural Integration of the Human Body*, now the Rolfing® method of Structural Integration. In 1971, Rolf founded The Rolf Institute of Structural Integration.[1]The Rolf Institute and a number of other schools, including the Guild for Structural Integration, Kinesis Myofascial Integration and Heller work Structural Integration, currently teach methods similar to the method presented by Rolf. **Theory and practice:** Rolf theorized that 'bound up' fascia (or connective tissue) often restricts opposing muscles from functioning in concert with one another, much in the way water, having crystallized, forms hard, unyielding ice. Her practice aimed to separate bound up fascia by deeply separating the fibers manually to loosen them and allow effective movement patterns. Rolf believed that an adequate knowledge of living human anatomy and hands-on training were required in order to safely negotiate the appropriate manipulations and depths necessary to free the bound-up fascia [citation needed]

Rolfers often prescribe a sequence of ten sessions to "balance and optimize both the structure (shape) and function (movement) of the entire body,"[5][6] usually beginning with the feet.[7] The theory is that "only by bringing peace 'from the ground up' can problems higher in the body be 'under-stood'".[7]During a Rolfing session, a client generally lies down and is guided through specific movements. The Rolfer manipulates the fascia until it can operate in conjunction with the muscles in a "normal" fashion.[6]

This takes place over a course of ten 75- to 90-minute sessions, with a specific goal for each session, and an overall goal of cumulative results.[8] Some clients find Rolfing painful, but Rolfing has evolved over the decades into a practice far more gentle than in its early origins.[9]

31.   pg. 118, From Wikipedia; **Jin Shin Do** ("The Way of the Compassionate Spirit") is a therapeutic massage technique developed in the 1970s by **Iona Marsaa Teeguarden derived from Jin Shin Jyutsu.**

It combines elements of Japanese acupressure, Chinese acupuncture, Orgone of Wilhelm Reich, Qigong, principles of Ericksonian psychotherapy, and Taoist philosophy, but uses its own specialized terminology. **Jin shin jitsu** (Jin shin jitsōō), *n.pr* a style of bodywork originating in Japan; promotes energetic movement through gentle pressure on multiple acupressure points. This is considered an inner bodywork modality because the techniques release emotional and spiritual—as well as physical—energies, From; Jonas: Mosby's Dictionary of Complementary and Alternative Medicine. (c) 2005, Elsevier.

32.   pg. 118, From Wikipedia: **Reiki** is a spiritual [1] developed in 1922 by Mikao Usui. After three weeks of fasting and meditating on Mount Kurama, in Japan, Usui claimed to receive the ability of "healing without energy depletion".[2] A portion of the practice, tenohira or palm healing, is used as a form of complementary and alternative medicine.[3][4] Tenohira is a technique whereby practitioners believe they are moving "healing energy" (a form of *ki*) through the palms.[5][6]

33.   pg. 118, From Wikipedia: **Emotional Freedom Techniques(EFT)** is a form of alternative psychotherapy, that purports to manipulate the body's energy by tapping on acupuncture while a specific traumatic memory is focused on, in order to alleviate a psychological problem. Critics have described the theory behind EFT as pseudoscientific and have suggested that any utility stems from its more traditional cognitive components, such as the placebo, distraction from negative thoughts, rather than from manipulation of meridians

34.   pg. 121, Colbin, Annemarie 'The Book of Whole Meals' New York, Ballantine Books 1983 pg. 23

35.   pg. 123, Colbin, Annemarie 'The Book of Whole Meals' New York, Ballantine Books 1983 pg. 23

36.   pg. 124, From Wikipedia: **A macrobiotic diet (or macrobiotics),** from the Greek "macro" (large, long) and "bios" (life), is a dietary regimen that involves eating grains as a staple food supplemented with other foodstuffs such as vegetables and beans, and avoiding the use of highly processed or refined foods. Macrobiotics also addresses the manner of eating by recommending against overeating and requiring that food be chewed thoroughly before swallowing. George Ohsawa brought his teaching to Europe from Japan.

Ohsawa was a Japanese philosopher, who was inspired to formalize macrobiotics by the teachings of Kaibara Ekiken, Andou Shōeki, Mizuno Namboku, and Sagen Ishizuka and his disciples Nishibata Manabu and Shojiro Goto. Ohsawa took his macrobiotic teachings to North America in the late 1950s. Macrobiotic education was spread in the United States by his students Herman Aihara, Cornelia Aihara, Michael Abehsera, Michio Kushi and Aveline Kushi, and in turn by their students.

Michio Kushi has been the most prominent of these teachers. Macrobiotics is considered an approach to life rather than a diet.

Some general guidelines for the diet are the following (it is also said that a macrobiotic diet varies greatly, depending on geographical and life circumstances):[7]

- Well chewed whole cereal grains, especially brown rice: 25–30%
- Vegetables: 30–40%
- Beans and legumes: 5–10%
- Miso soup: 5%
- Traditionally or naturally processed foods: 5–10%The remainder is composed of fish and seafood, seeds and nuts, seed and nut butters, seasonings, sweeteners, fruits, and beverages.
- Other naturally raised animal products may be included if needed during dietary transition or according to individual needs.

37.   pg. 126, From Wikipedia: **Donovan** (**Donovan Phillips Leitch**, born 10 May 1946, in Maryhill, Glasgow), is a Scottish singer-songwriter and guitarist. Emerging from the British folk scene, he developed an eclectic and distinctive style that blended folk, jazz, pop, psychedelia, and world music. 'There is a Mountain' Epic records 1967.

38.   pg. 126, From Wikipedia: The story of the **blind men and an elephant** originated from India. The story has been attributed to the Sufis, Jainists, Buddhists or Hindus, and has been used by all those groups. The version best-known in the West is the 19th Century poem by John Godfrey Saxe. Text is available under the Creative Commons Attribution-Share Alike License

39.   pg. 127, From Wikipedia: **Common knowledge** is that what "everybody knows", usually with reference to the community in which the term is used. The assertion that something is "common knowledge" is sometimes associated with the fallacy *argumentum ad populum* (Latin. "appeal to the people"). The fallacy essentially warns against assuming that just because everyone believes something is true does not make it so. Misinformation is easily introduced into rumors by intermediate messengers. Text is available under the Creative Commons Attribution-Share Alike License.

40.   pg. 130, From Wikipedia: *The Secret*, a film[1] produced by Prime Time, consists of a series of interviews related to the pseudo-scientific idea of "The Law of Attraction". Distributed through DVD, and online (through streaming media), the film and the subsequent publication of a book by the same name and of the same topic as the film.

41.   pg. 134, From Wikipedia: *Groundhog Day* is a 1993comedy film directed by Harold Ramis, starring Bill Murray and Andie MacDowell.It was written by Ramis and Danny Rubin, and based on a story by Rubin. In the film, Murray plays Phil Connors, an egocentric Pittsburgh TV weatherman who, during a hated assignment covering the annual Groundhog Day event (February 2) in Punxsutawney, finds himself repeating the same day over and over again. After indulging in all manner of hedonistic pursuits, then going through a suicidal streak, he begins to reexamine his life and priorities. In 2006, *Groundhog Day* was added to the United States National Film Registry as being deemed "culturally, historically, or aesthetically significant."

42. pg. 137, Tolle, Eckart 'Awakening to Your Life's Purpose' New York, Penguin Group, 2005

43. pg. 143, From Wikipedia: **Traditional Chinese Medicine,** also known as **TCM** (simplified Chinese: 中医; traditional Chinese: 中醫; pinyin: zhōng yī), includes a range of traditional medical practices originating in China. Although well accepted in the mainstream of medical care throughout East Asia, it is considered an alternative medical system in much of the western world. TCM practices include such treatments as herbal medicine (中药), acupuncture, dietary therapy, and both Tui na and Shiatsu massage. Qigong and Taijiquan are also closely associated with TCM.TCM claims to be rooted in meticulous observation of nature, the cosmos, and the human body, and to be thousands of years old. Major theories include those of Yin-yang, the Five Phases, the human body Channel system, Zang Fu organ theory, six confirmations, four layers, etc. Modern TCM was systematized in the 1950s under the People's Republic of China and Mao Zedong.

44. pg. 153, From Wikipedia: **Rudyard Kipling** (30 December1865 – 18 January1936) was a British author and poet, born in India. In 1907, he was awarded the Nobel Prize for Literature, making him the first English language writer to receive the prize, and he remains today its youngest-ever recipient. Poem; In the Neolithic Age 1895 stanza 5

45. pg. 156, From Wikipedia: **Golden ratio,** Text is available under the Creative Commons Attribution-Share Alike License.

46. pg. 160, From Wikipedia: **Royal Raymond Rife** (May 16, 1888 – August 5, 1971) was an American inventor known for his belief that he could observe and render inert a number of viruses which he thought were causal factors in several diseases, most notably cancer. The observations were made though a specially designed optical microscope, only five of which were ever constructed. Rife claimed that a "beam ray" device could devitalize the pathogens by inducing destructive resonances in their constituent chemicals.[1] Rife's claims could not be independently replicated, and active scientific interest in the devices had dissipated by the 1950s.Interest in Rife's claims was revived in some alternative medical spheres by the book *The Cancer Cure That Worked* (1987), which claimed that Rife's work was successful. The book also claimed that his cure for cancer was suppressed by a conspiracy headed by the American Medical Association.[2] After publication, a variety of devices bearing Rife's name were marketed as cures for diverse diseases such as cancer and AIDS.

47. pg. 160, From Wikipedia: **Electro acupuncture, also known as electro acupuncture according to Voll (EAV), electro dermal screening (EDS), bioelectric functions** diagnosis **(BFD), bio resonance therapy (BRT), or bio-energy regulatory technique (BER),** is a controversial alternative medicine method of using electro diagnostic devices to diagnose and treat "energy imbalance" often using homeopathic products, first used by Reinhold Voll by combining acupuncture with galvanometer in 1958.

48. pg. 162, 'GROUND HOG DAY LOOP' Refers to the repetitive life experience mirrored in the movie of the same name as a reflection of the cycle of karma and reincarnation.

49. pg. 162, From Wikipedia: *Root of all evil* is a figure of speech denoting something that causes all wickedness or suffering. By extension, it may be applied to any cause of serious problems.

The phrase derives from a saying attributed to Jesus in the Apostle Paul's First Epistle to Timothy in the New Testament: "The love of money is the root of all evil" (1 Timothy 6:10, KJV). The expression is commonly misquoted as simply "Money is the root of all evil".

50. pg. 166, From Wikipedia: A **deal with the Devil, pact with the Devil,** or **Faustian bargain** is a cultural motif widespread wherever belief in the Devil is vividly present, most familiar in the legend of Faust and the figure of Mephistopheles, but elemental to many Christian folktales. In the Aarne-Thompson typological catalogue, it lies in category AT 756B – "The devil's contract." According to traditional Christian belief in witchcraft, the pact is between a person and Satan or any other demon (or demons); the person offers his or her soul in exchange for diabolical favours. Those favours vary by the tale, but tend to include youth, knowledge, wealth, or power. It was also believed that some persons made this type of pact just as a sign of recognizing the Devil as their master, in exchange for nothing. Regardless, the bargain is a dangerous one, for the price of the Fiend's service is the wagerer's soul. The tale may have a moralizing end, with eternal damnation for the foolhardy venturer. Conversely it may have a comic twist, in which a wily peasant outwits the Devil, characteristically on a technical point.

51. pg. 166, From Wikipedia: Matthew 6:24–33 (King James Version "KJV"): No man can serve two masters: for either he will hate the one, and love the other; or else he will hold to the one, and despise the other. Ye cannot serve God and mammon. Therefore I say unto you, Take no thought for your life, what ye shall eat, or what ye shall drink; nor yet for your body, what ye shall put on. Is not the life more than meat, and the body than raiment? Behold the fowls of the air: for they sow not, neither do they reap, nor gather into barns; yet your heavenly Father feedeth them. Are ye not much better than they? Which of you by taking thought can add one cubit unto his stature? And why take ye thought for raiment? Consider the lilies of the field, how they grow; they toil not, neither do they spin: And yet I say unto you, that even Solomon in all his glory was not arrayed like one of these. Wherefore, if God so clothe the grass of the field, which today is, and tomorrow is cast into the oven, shall he not much more clothe you, O ye of little faith? Therefore take no thought, saying, What shall we eat? or, What shall we drink? or, Wherewithal shall we be clothed? (For after all these things do the Gentiles seek :) for your heavenly Father knoweth that ye have need of all these things. But seek ye first the kingdom of God, and his righteousness; and all these things shall be added unto you.

52. pg. 170, From Wikipedia: In quantum, the Heisenberg uncertainty principle states that certain pairs of physical properties, like position and momentum, cannot both be known to arbitrary precision. That is, the more precisely one property is known, the less precisely the other can be known. This statement has been interpreted in two different ways. According to Heisenberg its meaning is that it is impossible to determine simultaneously both the position and velocity of an electron or any other particle with any great degree of accuracy or certainty. According to others (for instance Ballentine [11]) this is not a statement about the limitations of a researcher's ability to measure particular quantities of a system, but it is a statement about the nature of the system itself as described by the equations of quantum mechanics.

53. pg. 170, Twitchell, Paul 'Approximate quote'. From Wikipedia: **Paul Twitchell** (born **John Paul Twitchell**) (October 22, 1908(?) - September 17, 1971) was an American spiritual writer, author and founder of the group known as Eckankar. He is accepted by the members of that group as the Mahanta, or Living ECK Master of his time.

He directed the development of the group through to the time of his death. His spiritual name is believed by Eckists (students of Eckankar) to be **Peddar Zaskq**.

54.   pg. 171, From Wikipedia: A **kōan** (pronounced /ˈkoʊ.ɑːn/; Chinese: 公案; pinyin: gōng-àn; Korean: gong'an; Vietnamese: công án) is a story, dialogue, question, or statement in the history and lore of Zen Buddhism, generally containing aspects that are inaccessible to rational understanding, yet may be accessible to intuition. A famous kōan is: "Two hands clap and there is a sound; what is the sound of one hand?" (oral tradition attributed to Hakuin Ekaku, 1686-1769, considered a reviver of the kōan tradition in Japan).

55.   pg. 171, From Wikipedia: A **freeze frame shot** is used when one shot is printed in a single frame several times, in order to make an interesting illusion of a still photograph. "Freeze frame" is also a drama medium term used in which, during a live performance, the actors/actresses will freeze at a particular, pre-meditated time, to enhance a particular scene, or to show an important moment in the play/ production[like a celebration]. The image can then be further enhanced by spoken word, in which each character tells their personal thoughts regarding the situation, giving the audience further insight into the meaning, plot or hidden story of the play/production/scene. This is known as thought tracking, another Drama Medium.

56. pg. 173, Morris, Elkan 'approximate quote from father'

57. pg. 174, Source; Bumper sticker, author anonymous

58. pg. 175,   Acronym original source unknown. **Following are several acronyms for F.E.A.R.** FEAR; First Encounter Assault Recon (gaming) FEAR; False Evidence Appearing Real FEAR; Forfeiture Endangers American Rights FEAR; Federal Employee Antidiscrimination and Retaliation Act of 2002 FEAR; False Expectations Appearing Real FEAR; Face Everything And Recover FEAR; Forget Everything And Run (polite form) FEAR; For Everything A Reason FEAR; Forget Everything and Remember FEAR; Finding Everything and Realizing (Ian Brown music video) FEAR; False Emotions Appearing Real FEAR; Failure Expected And Received FEAR; Future Events Appearing Real FEAR; Forgetting Everything is All Right FEAR; Finding Excuses and Reasons FEAR; Flexible Embodied Animat Architecture (language independent open-source project for the creation of portable AI) FEAR; False Expectations About Reality FEAR; Felines Enraged About Rodents (book - Ragweed) FEAR; Future Events Appear Real FEAR; Far East Adventure Racers (Hong Kong) FEAR; Frantic Effort to Avoid Reality

59. pg. 175,   Lee, Bruce: Movie; 'Silent Flute' renamed 'The Circle of Iron' From Wikipedia: **Circle of Iron** is a 1978 martial arts film co-written by Bruce Lee, who intended to star in the film himself, but he died before production. The film is also known as **The Silent Flute**, which was the original title of the story conceived by Bruce Lee, James Coburn, and Stirling Silliphant in 1969. After Lee's death in 1973, Silliphant and Stanley Mann completed the screenplay, and Lee's part was given to the Kung Fu television star, David Carradine. Many other well known character actors also had small roles in the film, including Roddy McDowall, Eli Wallach, and Christopher Lee. A martial artist rebel named Cord (played by Jeff Cooper) embarks on a quest for the Book of Enlightenment, which is kept by the mysterious Zetan (played by Christopher Lee). He must pass various trials along the way that educate him in Zen philosophy.

Among the characters that he runs across are a blind flute-player, a monkey chieftain, a death character, and the leader of a gypsy tribe (all played by David Carradine), who acts as a reluctant mentor to Cord. Some trials involve combat, while others involve riddles or encounters with unusual characters, such as a man (Eli Wallach) who has been standing in a barrel of oil for 10 years in an attempt to remove the lower half of his body so he is no longer distracted by his genitals. Cord successfully passes all trials and is able to view the *Book of Enlightenment.* He discovers that each page in the book is a mirror, showing him that the secret to enlightenment and all knowledge is already within himself. He then returns to the outside world to himself become a mentor for later seekers.

60. pg. 175, From Wikipedia: *Kung Fu* (1972–1975) is an American television series which starred David Carradine. It was created by Ed Spielman, directed and produced by Jerry Thorpe, and developed by Herman Miller, who was also a writer for, and co-producer of, the series. The show was preceded by a full length feature TV movie, an ABC "Movie of the Week", which was broadcast in 1972. *Kung Fu* follows the adventures of a Shaolin monk, Kwai Chang Caine [虔官昌 Qián Guānchāng] (portrayed by David Carradine as an adult, Keith Carradine as a teenager and Radames Pera as a young boy) who travels through the American Old West armed only with his skill in martial arts, as he seeks his half-brother, Danny Caine. Keye Luke (as the blind Master Po) and Philip Ahn (as Master Kan) were also members of the regular cast. David Chow, who was also a guest star in the series, acted as the technical and kung fu advisor, a role later undertaken by Kam Yuen. Overall series plot summary: Kwai Chang Caine (David Carradine) is the orphaned son of an American man and a Chinese woman in late 19th century China. After his maternal grandfather's death he is accepted for training at a Shaolin Monastery, where he grows up to become a Shaolin priest and martial arts expert. In the pilot episode Caine's beloved mentor and elder, Master Po, is murdered by the Emperor's nephew; outraged, Caine retaliates by killing the nephew. With a price on his head, Caine flees China to the western United States, where he seeks to find his family roots and, ultimately, his half-brother, Danny Caine. Although it is his intention to avoid notice, Caine's training and sense of social responsibility repeatedly force him out into the open, to fight for justice or protect the underdog. After each such encounter he must move on, both to avoid capture and prevent harm from coming to those he has helped. Flashbacks are often used to recall specific lessons from Caine's childhood training in the monastery from his teachers, the blind Master Po (Keye Luke) and Master Kan (Philip Ahn). Part of the appeal of the series was undoubtedly the emphasis laid, via the flashbacks, on the mental and spiritual power that Caine had gained from his rigorous training. In these flashbacks, Master Po calls his young student "Grasshopper" in reference to a scene in the pilot episode:

Master Po: Close your eyes. What do you hear?
Young Caine: I hear the water, I hear the birds.
Po: Do you hear your own heartbeat?
Caine: No.
Po: Do you hear the grasshopper which is at your feet?
Caine: Old man, how is it that you hear these things?
Po: Young man, how is it that you do not?[1]

61. pg. 185, From Wikipedia: The **Allegory of the Cave**, also commonly known as **Myth of the Cave**, **Metaphor of the Cave**, **The Cave Analogy**, **Plato's Cave** or the **Parable of the Cave**, is an allegory used by the Greek philosopher Plato in his work *The Republic* to illustrate "our nature in its education and want of education". (514a) The allegory of the cave is written as a fictional dialogue between Plato's teacher Socrates and Plato's brother Glaucon, at the beginning of Book VII (514a–520a).

363

Plato imagines a group of people who have lived chained in a cave all of their lives, facing a blank wall. The people watch shadows projected on the wall by things passing in front of a fire behind them, and begin to ascribe forms to these shadows. According to Plato, the shadows are as close as the prisoners get to seeing reality. He then explains how the philosopher is like a prisoner who is freed from the cave and comes to understand that the shadows on the wall are not constitutive of reality at all, as he can perceive the true form of reality rather than the mere shadows seen by the prisoners. The Allegory is related to Plato's Theory of Forms,[1] wherein Plato asserts that "Forms" (or "Ideas"), and not the material world of change known to us through sensation, possess the highest and most fundamental kind of reality. Only knowledge of the Forms constitutes real knowledge.[2] In addition, the allegory of the cave is an attempt to explain the philosopher's place in society. **In the Edge and Beyond, I identify "Forms", whether of things or "Ideas" as being bridges, to be mastered and released to lead to the "Formless".**

62. pg. 189, Sheldrake, Rupert 'The Hypothesis of a New Science of Life' Rochester, 1995 Park Street Press From Wikipedia: Rupert Sheldrake (born 28 June 1942) is a British former biochemist and plant physiologist who proposed a nonstandard account of morphogenesis and now researches in areas ranging from crystal melting points[1] to parapsychology. His books and papers stem from his theory of morphic resonance, and cover topics such as animal and plant development and behavior, memory, telepathy, perception and cognition in general.

63. pg. 191, Watson, Lyall 'Lifetide- A Biology of Unconscious' Coronet publishing, 1979. From Wikipedia: **Lyall Watson** (12 April 1939 - 25 June 2008) was a South botanist, zoologist, biologist, anthropologist, ethologist, and author of many new age books, among the most popular of which is the best seller *Supernature*. Lyall Watson tried to make sense of natural and supernatural phenomena in biological terms. He is credited with the first published use of the term Hundredth Monkey in his 1979 book, *Lifetide*. It is a hypothesis that aroused both interest and ire in the scientific community and continues to be a topic of discussion over a quarter century later.

64. pg. 192, Keyes, Ken Jr. 'The Hundredth Monkey'. From Wikipedia: **Ken Keyes, Jr.** (January 19, 1921, Atlanta, Georgia – December 20, 1995, Coos Bay, Oregon) was a personal growth author and lecturer, and the creator of the Living Love method, a self-help system. Married four times, Keyes wrote fifteen books on person growth and social consciousness issues, representing about four million copies distributed overall.

65. pg. 193, Keyes, Laurel Elizabeth ' The Creative Power of the Voice' Marina Del Rey, CA De Vorss and Company, Publisher 1973 **pg.21 Quote from Alfred Korzybski**. From Wikipedia: **Laurel Elizabeth Keyes** (died 1983) was an American author, lecturer and counselor. She is best-known for her early works on sound therapy and weight management. Biography: Keyes was a writer from an early age. Over the years, she wrote stories, articles and poetry for magazines and newspapers. She received her education in the transpersonal field from a variety of Eastern and Western sources, having started her studies in comparative religions and philosophy when she was 19. She lectured and conducted retreats for churches of all the major religions, and for more than 16 years lectured for adult education in the public school system. Her writings reflect a practical blending of popular in-depth methods of modern psychology and the ancient traditional teachings of metaphysics and philosophy. In 1952 Mrs. Keyes founded Overweight Overcomers International, one of the first self-help groups dedicated to problems of obesity, and wrote the book *How to Win the Losing Fight*, a weight-control guide that helped thousands to better health.

In 1963 she founded the Order of Fransisters and Brothers, a lay order following the outline of the well-known prayer beginning "Lord, make me an instrument" It is a non-profit, inter-religious movement, sponsoring silent retreats, study and research. Keyes' most popular book is her 1973 work *Toning: The Creative Power of the Voice*, which is cited by sound therapists. Her legacy also includes the Restorium, a chapel and retreat house in the mountains near Denver. Keyes resided in Denver, Colorado until her death in 1983. The sound and toning healing work of Keyes is again being carried on throughout the world in the integration of cymatics (sound) and light therapies. In the form of "giving voice" to bodily ailments, it has been integrated by Manhattan oncologist Dr. Mitchell L. Gaynor. Keyes' work has inspired Vibrations Heal, an on-going support and toning study group based in Burlington, Vermont. Vibrations Heal [1] teaches bi-weekly outreach meetings and seminar programs on the use of toning to maintain optimum health and restore health from many types of ailments and situations.

66. pg. 194, Keyes, Laurel Elizabeth 'Toning The Creative Power of the Voice' Marina Del Rey, CA De Vorss and Company, Publisher 1973 **pg. 5 Quote**

67. pg. 194, Keyes, Laurel Elizabeth 'Toning The Creative Power of the Voice' Marina Del Rey, CA De Vorss and Company, Publisher 1973 **pg. 5 Quote from Bach, Marcus, PhD., 'The Inner Ecstasy'**, Abingdon Press, Nashville, Tenn. 1969.

68. pg. 201, From Wikipedia: The **Gaia hypothesis** is an ecological hypothesis proposing that the biosphere and the physical components of the Earth (atmosphere, cryosphere, hydrosphere and lithosphere) are closely integrated to form a complex that maintains the climatic and biogeochemical conditions on Earth in a preferred homeostasis. Originally proposed by James Lovelock as the earth feedback hypothesis, [1] it was named the Gaia Hypothesis after the Greek of Earth.[2]

The hypothesis is frequently described as viewing the Earth as a single organism. Lovelock and other supporters of the idea now call it **Gaia theory,** regarding it as a scientific theory and not mere hypothesis, since they believe it has passed predictive tests.[3]

69. pg. 206, Dass, Ram 'Remember Be Here Now' New York, Crown Publishing 1978 Hanuman Foundation. From Wikipedia: **Richard Alpert** (born April 6, 1931), also known as **Baba Ram Dass,** is a contemporary spiritual teacher who wrote the 1971 bestseller *Remember Be Here*. He is well known for his personal and professional association with Timothy Leary at Harvard in the early 1960s. He is also known for his travels to India and his relationship with the Hindu guru Neem Karoli Baba.

70. pg. 209, *Reynolds, Malvina: Song 'Magic Penny' from album Reynolds... Sings The Truth* (1968) on Columbia, CS 9414. From Wikipedia: Malvina Reynolds (born as Malvina Milder on August 23, 1900, died March 17, 1978) was an American folk/blues singer-songwriter and political, probably best known for writing the song "Little Boxes".[1]

71. pg. 218, From Wikipedia: **Epictetus** (Greek: Ἐπίκτητος; AD 55–AD 135) was a Greek Stoic philosopher. He was probably born a slave at Hierapolis, Phrygia (present day Pamukkale, Turkey), and lived in Rome until his exile to Nicopolis in northwestern Greece, where he lived most of his life and died.

His teachings were notated and published by his pupil Arrian in his *Discourses*. Philosophy, he taught, is a way of life and not just a theoretical discipline.

To Epictetus, all external events are determined by fate, and are thus beyond our control, but we can accept whatever happens calmly and dispassionately. Individuals, however, are responsible for their own actions which they can examine and control through rigorous self-discipline. Suffering arises from trying to control what is uncontrollable, or from neglecting what is within our power. As part of the universal city that is the universe, human beings have a duty of care to all fellow humans. The person who followed these precepts would achieve happiness

72. pg. 220, From Wikipedia: ***Ghostbusters*** (titled on-screen as *Ghost Busters*) is a 1984 American science comedy film written by co-stars Dan Aykroyd and Harold Ramis about three eccentric New York City parapsychologists-turned-ghost exterminators. The film was released in the United States on June 8, 1984 and like several films of the era, teamed Aykroyd and/or Ramis with headliner Bill Murray.

73. pg. 226, "QUOTE" from **song.** From Wikipedia: The **Boom Boom Satellites** (ブンブンサテライツ, *Bun Bun Sateraitsu?*) are a Japanese electronic duo consisting of guitarist and vocalist Michiyuki Kawashima and bassist and programmer Masayuki Nakano. While their music can be mostly classified as big beat or nu skool breaks with heavy jazz influences, they are famous for the heavy usage of electric in their music, and the final product often has a strong rock or punk flavor. They are currently signed to Sony Music, with whom they have released all of their albums in Japan.

74. pg. 231, From Wikipedia: ***Men are from Mars, Women are from Venus*** (published in May 1992) is a book by John Gray offering many suggestions for improving men-women relationships in couples by understanding the communication style and emotional needs of the opposite gender. It spawned a series of follow-on books expanding on specific situations (see below). The book, as suggested by the title, asserts the notion that men and women are as different as beings from other planets. Gray adopts this metaphor as the central theme of all his books and seminars, likening men and women to the classical Roman god Mars and goddess Venus as ideal types. In contrast to some psychologists (and feminists) who emphasize similarities between the sexes, Gray writes almost exclusively about differences. Gray says that his "Martians" and "Venusians" are only stereotypes and cannot be applied blindly to individuals. An example of the theories it offers is that women complain about problems because they want their problems to be acknowledged, while men complain about problems because they are asking for solutions. Other concepts in the book are the difference between women and men's point systems and how they react under stress.

75.pg. 234, From Wikipedia: **Shamanism** (/ˈʃɑːmən/ *SHAH-mən* or /ˈʃeɪmən/ *SHAY-mən*) is a practice that involves a practitioner reaching altered states of consciousness in order to encounter and interact with the spirit world and channel these transcendental energies into this world.[2]

A shaman is a person regarded as having access to, and influence in, the world of benevolent and malevolent spirits, who typically enters into a trance state during a ritual, and practices divination and healing.[3]The term "shamanism" is currently often used as an umbrella term referring to a variety of spiritual practices, although it was first applied to the ancient religion of the Turks and Mongols, as well as those of the neighboring Tungusic and Samoyedic-speaking peoples. The word "shaman" originates from the Evenk language (Tungusic) of North Asia and was introduced to the west after Russian forces conquered the shamanistic Khanate of Kazan in 1552.

Upon learning more about religious traditions across the world, western scholars also described similar magico-religious practices found within the indigenous religions of other parts of Asia, Africa, Australasia and the Americas as shamanism.

Various historians have argued that shamanism also played a role in many of the pre-Christian religions of Europe, and that shamanic elements may have survived in popular culture right through to the Early Modern period. Various archaeologists and historians of religion have also suggested that shamanism may have been a dominant pre-religious practice for humanity during the Palaeolithic. Mircea Eliade writes, "A first definition of this complex phenomenon, and perhaps the least hazardous, will be: shamanism = ‹technique of religious ecstasy'."[4] Shamanism encompasses the premise that shamans are intermediaries or messengers between the human world and the spirit worlds. Shamans are said to treat ailments/illness by mending the soul. Alleviating traumas affecting the soul/spirit restores the physical body of the individual to balance and wholeness. The shaman also enters supernatural realms or dimensions to obtain solutions to problems afflicting the community. Shamans may visit other worlds/dimensions to bring guidance to misguided souls and to ameliorate illnesses of the human soul caused by foreign elements. The shaman operates primarily within the spiritual world, which in turn affects the human world. The restoration of balance results in the elimination of the ailment.[4] Shamanic beliefs and practices have attracted the interest of scholars from a wide variety of disciplines, including anthropologists, archaeologists, historians, religious studies scholars and psychologists. Hundreds of books and academic papers on the subject have been produced,[citation needed] with a peer-reviewed academic journal being devoted to the study of shamanisms.[citation d In the 20th century, many westerners involved in the counter-cultural movement adopted magico-religious practices influenced by indigenous shamanisms from across the world, creating the Neoshamanic movement.

76. pg. 234, From Wikipedia: An **entheogen** ("generating the divine within») [4] is a psychoactive substance used in a religious, shamanic, or spiritual context. [5] Entheogens can supplement many diverse practices for transcendence, and revelation, including meditation, psychonautics, psychedelic and visionary art, psychedelic therapy, and magic. Entheogens have been used in a ritualized context for thousands of years; their religious significance is well established in anthropological and modern evidences. Examples of traditional entheogens include: peyote, psilocybin mushrooms, uncured tobacco, cannabis, ayahuasca, Salvia divinorum, Tabernanthe iboga, Ipomoea tricolor, and Amanita muscaria. With the advent of organic chemistry, there now exist many synthetic substances with similar psychoactive properties, many derived from these plants. Many pure active compounds with psychoactive properties have been isolated from these organisms and chemically synthesized, including mescaline, psilocybin, DMT, salvinorin A, ibogaine, ergotamine, and muscimol, respectively. Semisynthetic (e.g. LSD is usually derived from ergotamine) and synthetic substances (e.g. DPT used by the Temple of the True Inner Light and 2C-B used by the Sangoma) have also been developed.[6] Entheogens may be compounded through the work of a shaman or apothecary in a tea, admixture, or potion like ayahuasca or bhang. More broadly, the term *entheogen* is used to refer to any psychoactive substances when used for their religious or spiritual effects, whether or not in a formal religious or traditional structure. This terminology is often chosen to contrast with recreational use of the same substances. Studies such as the Marsh Chapel Experiment have documented reports of spiritual experiences from participants who were administered psychoactive substances in controlled trials.[7] Ongoing research is limited due to widespread drug prohibition; however, some countries have legislation that allows for traditional entheogen use.

77. pg. 236, From Wikipedia; 1990 - *Sacred Mirrors: The Visionary Art of Alexander Grey* (Alex Grey) (Inner Traditions - Bear & Company) ISBN 0892813148. **Alex Grey** (born November 29, 1953) is an American artist specializing in spiritual and psychedelic art (or visionary art) that is sometimes associated with the New Age movement. Grey is a Vajrayana practitioner.

His body of work spans a variety of forms including performance art, process art, installation art, sculpture, visionary art, and painting. Grey is a member of the Integral Institute. He is also on the board of advisors for the Center for Cognitive Liberty and Ethics, and is the Chair of Wisdom University's Sacred Art Department. He and his wife Allyson Grey are the co-founders of the Chapel of Sacred Mirrors, a non-profit institution supporting Visionary Culture in New York City.

78. pg. 244, From Wikipedia: "**Let It Be**" is a song by The Beatles, released in March 1970 as a single, and (in an alternate mix) as the title track of their album *Let It Be*. Although credited to Lennon/McCartney it is generally accepted to be a Paul McCartney composition.

79. pg. 245, From Wikipedia: *The Matrix* is a 1999 American–Australian science fiction action film written and directed by The Wachowski Brothers, and starring Keanu Reeves, Laurence Fishburne, Carrie-Anne Moss, Joe Pantoliano, and Hugo Weaving. It depicts a dystopian future in which reality as perceived by most humans is actually a simulated reality called "the Matrix", created by sentient machines to subdue the human population, while their bodies› heat and electrical activity are used as an energy source.

Computer programmer «Neo" learns this truth and is drawn into a rebellion against the machines, which involves other people who have been freed from the "dream world". *The Matrix* is known for popularizing a visual effect known as "bullet time", in which the heightened perception of certain characters is represented by allowing the action within a shot to progress in slow-motion while the camera's viewpoint appears to move through the scene at normal speed. The film is an example of the cyberpunk science fiction genre.[3]

It contains numerous references to philosophical and religious ideas, and prominently pays homage to works such as Plato's Allegory of the Cave, Jean Baudrillard's *Simulacra and Simulation*[4] and Lewis Carroll's *Alice's Adventures in Wonderland*. The Wachowskis' approach to action scenes drew upon their admiration for Japanese animation[5] and martial arts films, and the film's use of fight choreographers and wire fu techniques from Hong Kong action cinema was influential upon subsequent Hollywood action film productions. *The Matrix* was first released in the United States on March 31, 1999, and grossed over $460 million worldwide. It was generally well-received by critics,[6][7] and won four Academy Awards as well as other accolades including BAFTA Awards and Saturn Awards. Reviewers praised *The Matrix* for its innovative visual effects, cinematography and its entertainment. The film's premise was both criticized for being derivative of earlier science fiction works, and praised for being intriguing. The action also polarized critics, some describing it as impressive, but others dismissing it as a trite distraction from an interesting premise. Despite this, the film has since appeared in lists of the greatest science fiction films,[8][9][10] and in 2012, was added to the National Film Registry for preservation.[11] The success of the film led to the release of two feature film sequels, both written and directed by the Wachowskis, *The Matrix Reloaded* and *The Matrix Revolutions*. The *Matrix* franchise was further expanded through the production of comic books, video games, and animated short films in which the Wachowskis were heavily involved.

The series depicts a <u>dystopia</u> in which Earth is dominated by <u>sentient machines</u> that were created early in the 21st century and rebelled against humanity. At one point, humans attempted to block out the machines› source of <u>solar power</u> by covering the sky in thick, stormy clouds. However, the machines devised a way to extract humans' <u>bioelectricity</u> and <u>thermal energy</u> by growing people in pods, while their minds are kept under control by cybernetic implants connecting them to a <u>simulated reality</u> called the Matrix. The virtual reality world simulated by the Matrix resembles human civilization around the turn of the 21st century (this time period was chosen because it is supposedly the pinnacle of human civilization).

The majority of the stories in the *Matrix* franchise take place in a vast <u>unnamed megacity</u>. This environment is practically indistinguishable from reality (although scenes set within the Matrix are presented on-screen with a bias toward the color green), and the majority of humans connected to the Matrix are unaware of its true nature. Most of the central characters in the series are able to gain <u>superhuman</u> abilities within the Matrix by using their understanding of its true nature to manipulate its <u>physical laws</u>. The virtual world is first introduced in *The Matrix*. The *Animatrix* short film "The Second Renaissance" and the short comic "Bits and Pieces of Information" show how the initial conflict between humans and machines came about, and how and why the Matrix was first developed. Its history and purpose are further explained in *The Matrix Reloaded*.

80. pg. 246, From Wikipedia: **Avatar** is a 2009 American[8][9] epic science fiction action film directed, written, co-produced, and co-edited by James Cameron, and starring Sam Worthington, Zoe Saldana, Stephen Lang, Michelle Rodriguez, Joel David Moore, Giovanni Ribisi, and Sigourney Weaver. The film is set in the mid-22nd century, when humans are mining a precious mineral called unobtanium on Pandora, a lush habitable moon of a gas giant in the Alpha Centauri star system.[10][11][12] The expansion of the mining colony threatens the continued existence of a local tribe of Na'vi – a humanoid species indigenous to Pandora. The film›s title refers to a genetically engineered Na'vi body with the mind of a remotely located human, and is used to interact with the natives of Pandora.[13] Development of *Avatar* began in 1994, when Cameron wrote an 80-page treatment for the film.[14][15] Filming was supposed to take place after the completion of Cameron's 1997 film *Titanic*, for a planned release in 1999,[16] but according to Cameron, the necessary technology was not yet available to achieve his vision of the film. [17] Work on the language of the film's extraterrestrial beings began in summer 2005, and Cameron began developing the screenplay and fictional universe in early 2006.[18][19] Following the film's success, Cameron signed with 20th Century Fox to produce three sequels, making *Avatar* the first of a planned tetralogy. [33] Plot: By 2154, humans have severely depleted Earth's natural resources. The Resources Development Administration (RDA) mines for a valuable mineral – unobtanium – on Pandora, a densely forested habitable moon orbiting the gas giant Polyphemus in the Alpha Centauri star system.[12] Pandora, whose atmosphere is poisonous to humans, is inhabited by the Na›vi, 10-foot tall (3.0 m), blue-skinned, sapient humanoids[34] who live in harmony with nature and worship a mother goddess called Eywa. To explore Pandora›s biosphere, scientists use Na'vi-human hybrids called "avatars", operated by genetically matched humans; Jake Sully, a paraplegic former marine, replaces his deceased twin brother as an operator of one. Dr. Grace Augustine, head of the Avatar Program, considers Sully an inadequate replacement but accepts his assignment as a bodyguard. While protecting the avatars of Grace and scientist Norm Spellman as they collect biological data, Jake's avatar is attacked by a thanator and flees into the forest, where he is rescued by Neytiri, a female Na'vi. Witnessing an auspicious sign, she takes him to her clan, whereupon Neytiri's mother Mo'at, the clan's spiritual leader, orders her daughter to initiate Jake into their society.

Colonel Miles Quaritch, head of RDA›s private security force, promises Jake that the company will restore his legs if he gathers intelligence about the Na'vi and the clan's gathering place, a giant arboreal called Hometree,[35] on grounds that it stands above the richest deposit of unobtanium in the area. When Grace learns of this, she transfers herself, Jake, and Norm to an outpost. Over three months, Jake grows to sympathize with the natives. After Jake is initiated into the tribe, he and Neytiri choose each other as mates, and soon afterward, Jake reveals his change of allegiance when he attempts to disable a bulldozer that threatens to destroy a sacred Na›vi site.

When Quaritch shows a video recording of Jake's attack on the bulldozer to Administrator Parker Selfridge,[36] and another in which Jake admits that the Na'vi will never abandon Hometree, Selfridge orders Hometree destroyed. Despite Grace›s argument that destroying Hometree could damage the biological neural network native to Pandora, Selfridge gives Jake and Grace one final chance to convince the Na'vi to evacuate before commencing the attack. While trying to warn the Na'vi, Jake confesses to being a spy and the Na'vi take him and Grace captive. Seeing this, Quaritch's men destroy Hometree, killing Neytiri's father (the clan chief) and many others. Mo'at frees Jake and Grace, but they are detached from their avatars and imprisoned by Quaritch's forces. Pilot Trudy Chacón, disgusted by Quaritch's brutality, carries them to Grace's outpost, but during the escape, Quaritch fires at them, hitting Grace.

To regain the Na'vi's trust, Jake connects his mind to that of Toruk, a dragonlike predator feared and honoured by the Na'vi. Jake finds the refugees at the sacred Tree of Souls and pleads with Mo'at to heal Grace. The clan attempts to transfer Grace from her human body into her avatar with the aid of the Tree of Souls, but she dies before the process can complete. Supported by the new chief Tsu›tey, who acts as Jake›s translator, Jake speaks to unite the clan and tells them to gather all of the clans to battle against the RDA. Noticing the impending gathering, Quaritch organizes a pre-emptive strike against the Tree of Souls, believing that its destruction will demoralize the natives. On the eve of battle, Jake prays to Eywa, via a neural connection to the Tree of Souls, to intercede on behalf of the Na›vi. During the subsequent battle, the Na›vi suffer heavy casualties, including Tsu›tey and Trudy; but are rescued when Pandoran wildlife unexpectedly join the attack and overwhelm the humans, which Neytiri interprets as Eywa's answer to Jake›s prayer. Then Jake destroys a makeshift bomber before it can reach the Tree of Souls; Quaritch escapes from his own damaged aircraft, wearing an AMP suit and breaks open the avatar link unit containing Jake›s human body, exposing it to Pandora's poisonous atmosphere. Quaritch then prepares to slit the throat of Jake›s avatar, but Neytiri kills Quaritch and saves Jake from suffocation. With the exceptions of Jake, Norm, Max and a few other scientists, all humans are expelled from Pandora and sent back to Earth, after which Jake is transferred permanently into his avatar with the aid of the Tree of Souls.

81. pg. 248, From Wikipedia: **Ecology** (from Greek: οἶκος, «house»; -λογία, «study of»[A]) is the scientific study of interactions among organisms and their environment, such as the interactions organisms have with each other and with their abiotic environment. Topics of interest to ecologists include the diversity, distribution, amount (biomass), number (population) of organisms, as well as competition between them within and among ecosystems. Ecosystems are composed of dynamically interacting parts including organisms, the communities they make up, and the non-living components of their environment. Ecosystem processes, such as primary production, pedogenesis, nutrient cycling, and various niche construction activities, regulate the flux of energy and matter through an environment. These processes are sustained by organisms with specific life history traits, and the variety of organisms is called biodiversity. Biodiversity, which refers to the varieties of species, genes, and ecosystems, enhances certain ecosystem services.

Ecology is an interdisciplinary field that includes biology and Earth science.The word "ecology" ("Ökologie") was coined in 1866 by the German scientist Ernst Haeckel (1834–1919). Ancient Greek philosophers such as Hippocrates and Aristotle laid the foundations of ecology in their studies on natural history. Modern ecology transformed into a more rigorous science in the late 19th century. Evolutionary concepts on adaptation and natural selection became cornerstones of modern ecological theory. Ecology is not synonymous with environment, environmentalism, natural history, or environmental science. It is closely related to evolutionary biology, genetics, and ethology. An understanding of how biodiversity affects ecological function is an important focus area in ecological studies. Ecologists seek to explain:

- Life processes, interactions and adaptations
- The movement of materials and energy through living communities
- The successional development of ecosystems, and
- The abundance and distribution of organisms and biodiversity in the context of the environment.

Ecology is a human science as well. There are many practical applications of ecology in conservation biology, wetland management, natural resource management (agroecology, agriculture, forestry, agroforestry, fisheries), city planning (urban ecology), community health, economics, basic and applied science, and human social interaction (human ecology). Organisms and resources compose ecosystems which, in turn, maintain biophysical feedback mechanisms that moderate processes acting on living (biotic) and nonliving (abiotic) components of the planet. Ecosystems sustain life-supporting functions and produce natural capital like biomass production (food, fuel, fiber and medicine), the regulation of climate, global biogeochemical cycles, water filtration, soil formation, erosion control, flood protection and many other natural features of scientific, historical, economic, or intrinsic value.

82. pg. 250, From Wikipedia: The **Maya calendar** is a system of calendars used in pre-Columbian Mesoamerica, and in many modern communities in highland Guatemala[1] and in Veracruz, Oaxaca and Chiapas, Mexico.[2] The essentials of the Maya calendar are based upon a system which had been in common use throughout the region, dating back to at least the 5th century BCE. It shares many aspects with calendars employed by other earlier Mesoamerican civilizations, such as the Zapotec and Olmec, and contemporary or later ones such as the Mixtec and Aztec calendars.[3] Although the Mesoamerican calendar did not originate with the Maya, their subsequent extensions and refinements of it were the most sophisticated.[citation needed] Along with those of the Aztecs, the Maya calendars are the best-documented and most completely understood.[citation needed]By the Maya mythological tradition, as documented in Colonial Yucatec accounts and reconstructed from Late Classic and Post classic inscriptions, the deity Itzamna is frequently credited with bringing the knowledge of the calendar system to the ancestral Maya, along with writing In general and other foundational aspects of Maya culture.[4]

83. pg. 252, From Wikipedia: **LGBT** is an initialism that stands for **lesbian, gay, bisexual, and transgender**. In use since the 1990s, the term is an adaptation of the initialism **LGB**, which itself started replacing the term *gay* when in reference to the community beginning in the mid-to-late 1980s,[1] as many felt the term *gay community* did not accurately represent all those to whom it referred.[2]

371

The initialism has become mainstream as a self-designation and has been adopted by the majority of sexuality and gender identity-based community centers and media in the United States and some other English-speaking countries.[3][4] It is also used in some other countries in whose languages the initialism is meaningful, such as France. The initialism LGBT is intended to emphasize a diversity of sexuality and gender identity-based cultures and is sometimes used to refer to anyone who is non-heterosexual or non-cisgender instead of exclusively to people who are lesbian, gay, bisexual, or transgender.[2][5]

To recognize this inclusion, a popular variant adds the letter Q for those who identify as queer and/or are questioning their sexual identity as *LGBTQ*, recorded since 1996.[6] On the one hand, some intersex people who want to be included in LGBT groups suggest an extended initialism *LGBTI* (recorded since 1999[7]).[8] This initialism "LGBTI" is used in all parts of «The Activists Guide» of the Yogyakarta Principles in Action.[9] Furthermore, the initialism *LGBTIH* has seen use in India to encompass the hijra third gender identity and the related subculture.[10] More recently the catch-all term "Gender and Sexual Diversity" **GSD** has been proposed.[11] Whether or not LGBT people openly identify themselves may depend on whether they live in a discriminatory environment, as well as the status of LGBT rights where one lives.[12]

84. pg. 254, From Wikipedia: **Tantra**[note 1] is the name given by scholars to a style of meditation and ritual which arose in India no later than the fifth century AD.[1] The earliest documented use of the word «Tantra» is in the Rigveda (X.71.9).[2] Tantra has influenced the Hindu, Bön, Buddhist, and Jain traditions and spread with Buddhism to East and Southeast Asia.[3] Tantric path[edit] *For Tibetan Buddhist ideas, see Anuttarayoga Tantra.* Long training is generally required to master Tantric methods. Pupils are typically initiated by a guru. A number of techniques are used as aids for meditation and achieving spiritual power:

- Yoga, including breathing techniques and postures (*asana*), is employed to subject the body to the control of the will.
- Mudras, or gestures
- Mantras: Syllables, words and phrases
- Mandalas
- Yantras: Symbolic diagrams of forces at work in the universe
- Identification with deities

The process of sublimation consists of three phases:
1. Purification
2. Elevation
3. «Reaffirmation of identity in pure consciousness»[38]

Sexual rites [edit] Although equated with Tantra in the West, sexual rites were historically practiced by a minority of sects. For practicing groups, maithuna progressed into psychological symbolism.[50] Origins [edit] According to White, the sexual rites of Vamamarga may have emerged from early Hindu Tantra as a means of catalyzing biochemical transformations in the body to facilitate heightened states of awareness.[50] These constitute an offering to Tantric deities. Religious aims [edit] See also: Neotantra Later developments in the rite emphasize the primacy of bliss and divine union, which replace the bodily connotations of earlier forms.[50] When enacted as enjoined by the Tantras, the ritual culminates in an experience of awareness for both participants.

Tantric texts specify that **sex** has three distinct purposes: procreation, pleasure and liberation. Those seeking liberation eschew orgasm in favor of a higher form of **ecstasy**. Several sexual rituals are recommended and practiced, involving elaborate preparatory and purification rites. The sexual act balances energies in the **pranic ida** and **pingala** channels in the bodies of both participants. The **sushumna nadi** is awakened, and **kundalini** rises within it. This culminates in *samadhi*, where the individual personality and identity of each participant is dissolved in **cosmic consciousness**. Tantrics understand these acts on multiple levels. The male and female participants are conjoined physically, representing *Shiva* and *Shakti* (the male and female principles). A fusion of *Shiva* and *Shakti* energies takes place, resulting in a unified energy.

85. pg. 259, From Wikipedia: The phrase "**Earth Changes**" was coined by the American psychic Edgar Cayce to refer to the belief that the world will soon enter on a series of cataclysmic events causing major alterations in human life on the planet. This includes «natural events» (such as major earthquakes, the melting of the polar ice caps, a pole shift of the planetary axis, major weather events, solar flares and so on[1]) as well as huge changes of the local and global social, economical and political systems. Cayce [edit]. Cayce himself also made many prophesies of cataclysmic events involving the whole planet.[2][3] He claimed the polar axis would shift and that many areas that are now land would again become ocean floor, and that Atlantis would rise from the sea.[3] The belief that the California coast would slip into the sea—a common feature of Earth Changes predictions—originated with Cayce›s alleged prophecies.[citation needed] In more recent times, self-proclaimed psychic Gordon-Michael Scallion has issued a variety of prophecies centering on the concept of "Earth Changes" and publishes a monthly newsletter, *The Earth Changes Report*.[4] New Age [edit] Cayce's term has been taken up in certain segments of the New Age movement,[5] often associated with other predictions by people claiming to have psychic abilities.[6] Belief in Earth changes is also found among Native Americans, some of whom refer to the concept as "the Great Purification."[7] These beliefs have occasionally been associated with Christian millennialism and beliefs about UFOs.[1] Some New Age adherents believe that Earth changes will preface a "Golden Age" of spirituality and world peace.[2][5] Reception and interpretation [edit] Prophecies of Earth changes have been described as a form of pseudoscience, in which terminology and ideas borrowed from science are used to rationalize non-scriptural apocalyptical thought based on visionary experiences.[6] David Spangler, a leader of the Findhorn Foundation spiritual community, described prophecies of Earth changes as an expression of collective fear and anger, rather than as foretelling of actual future events.[8]

86. pg. 265, From Wikipedia: **Warp drive** is a faster-than-light (FTL) propulsion system in the universe of many science settings, most notably Star Trek. A spacecraft equipped with a warp drive may travel at velocities greater than that of light by many orders of magnitude, whilst circumventing the relativistic problem of time. Some of the other fictions in which warp drive technology is featured include: Stars!, EVE Online, StarCraft, Darkspace, Starship Troopers, and Red Dwarf.

In contrast to many other fictional FTL technologies, such as a "jump drive" or the Infinite Improbability Drive, the warp drive does not permit instantaneous travel between two points; instead, warp drive technology creates an artificial "bubble" of normal space-time that surrounds the spacecraft (as opposed to entering a separate realm or dimension like hyperspace). Consequently, spacecraft at warp velocity can continue to interact with objects in normal space.

The idea of warping space as a means of propulsion has enjoyed theoretical study by physicists such as Miguel Alcubierre, who has designed his own hypothetical drive.[1][2] However, an approach that may be facilitated by our present level of technological advancement has yet to be proposed.

87. pg. 268, From Wikipedia: ***The Road to El Dorado*** is a 2000 American animated adventure musical comedy film directed by Eric "Bibo" Bergeron and Will Finn, with additional sequences by Don Paul and David Silverman, starring Kevin Kline, Kenneth Branagh, and Rosie Pérez, and produced by DreamWorks. The soundtrack features songs by Elton John and Tim Rice, as well as composer Hans Zimmer, the music team from Disney's *The Lion King.* The movie begins in 16th century Seville, Spain, and tells about two men named Tulio and Miguel.

During a dice game using loaded dice, they win a map that supposedly shows the location of El Dorado, the legendary city of gold in the New World. However, their cheating is soon discovered and as a result, they end up as stowaways on Hernán Cortés' fleet to conquer Mexico.

They are discovered, but manage to escape in a boat with Cortés' prize war horse and eventually discover the hidden city of El Dorado where they are mistaken for gods. It is inspired by Rudyard Kipling's *The Man Who Would Be King.*

88. pg. 273, From Wikipedia: **Burning Man** is a week-long annual event held in the Black Rock Desert in northern Nevada, in the United States. The event begins on the last Monday in August, and ends on the first Monday in September, which coincides with the American Labor Day holiday. It takes its name from the ritual burning of a large wooden effigy, which is set alight on Saturday evening. The event is described as an experiment in community, art, radical self-expression, and radical self-reliance.[1][2][3][4] Burning Man is organized by Black Rock City, LLC. In 2010, 51,515 people attended Burning Man.[5] 2011 attendance was capped at 50,000 participants and the event sold out on July 24.[6] In April 2011, Larry Harvey announced that the organization had begun the process of transitioning management of Burning Man over to a new non-profit organization called the «Burning Man Project».

89. pg. 273, From **EarthDance.org homepage: A Global Collaboration Since 1997**; Earthdance is the world's largest synchronized music and dance festival for peace. Since its inception, Earthdance has been held on over 500 locations in 80 countries with all events simultaneously joining together in the Prayer for Peace - a powerful moment of coherent intention.

Each public earthdance event gives 50% of their profits to a charity that falls into one of the following categories:-The Welfare of Children & Urban Youth, Indigenous Peoples & Cultures, International Relief and Development, Environmental Sustainability & Protection, Organizations that help Promote Peace. Earthdance occurs annually every September in recognition of the United Nations International Day of Peace with the intention to build a Culture of Peace.

90. pg. 273, From Wikipedia: **Techno** is a form of electronic (EDM)[1] that emerged in Detroit, Michigan, USA during the mid to late 1980s. The first recorded use of the word *techno*, in reference to a genre of music, was in 1988.[2][3] Many styles of techno now exist, but Detroit techno is seen as the foundation upon which a number of subgenres have been built.[4] The initial take on techno arose from the melding of Eurocentric synthesizer-based music with various African American styles such as Chicago house, funk, electro, and electric. Added to this is the influence of futuristic and fictional themes[5] that are relevant to life in American late capitalist society—particularly the book *The Third Wave* by Alvin Toffler.[6][7] Pioneering producer Juan Atkins cites Toffler's phrase "techno rebels" as inspiring him to use the word *techno* to describe the musical style he helped to create. This unique blend of influences aligns techno with the aesthetic referred to as afro-futurism. To producers such as Derrick May, the transference of spirit from the body to the machine is often a central preoccupation; essentially an expression of technological spirituality.[8][9] In this manner: "*techno dance music defeats what Adorno saw as the alienating effect of mechanization on the modern consciousness*".[10] Music journalists and fans of techno are generally selective in their use of the term; so a clear distinction can be made between sometimes related but often qualitatively different styles, such as tech house and trance. "Techno" is also commonly confused with generalized descriptors, such as electronic music and dance music.[11][12][13] **Progressive electronic dance music** usually refers to differentiate various offshoot styles of electronic dance music (EDM) from their parent styles, which include trance, house music, breakbeat and GRP fusion. Most electronic dance music tracks released today contain features that are relatively easy for DJs to beat match records together partly for that reason.

Unlike the song structures of genres like hard house or Hi-NRG, the peaks and troughs in a progressive dance track tend to be more complex. Layering has come to refer to the structure of a track with more gradual changes, though there are other uses for the term: *progressive trance* usually refers to a type of trance music that features a less prominent lead melody and focuses more on atmosphere, and in the case of progressive house, the term "progressive" can also refer to the style's willingness to bring in new elements to the genre. These elements can be a variety of sounds, such as a guitar loop, computer generated noises, or other elements typical of other genres. **Progressive house;** is a style of house music that is noted for musical progression within melodies and bass lines. The term was coined by Mixmag editor Dom Phillips. It has similar elements to both electro-house and trance. It has its origins in Great Britain in the early 1990s, with the output of Guerilla Records and Leftfield's first singles (particularly "Song of Life"). The music itself was produced with the 4-to-4 beat of house music and deeper dub-influenced bass lines, with greater emphasis on emotion before structural considerations. Often, it featured elements from many different genres mixed together. *Song of Life*, for instance, has a trip-hop like down-pitched breakbeat and a high-energy Roland TB riff at various stages. In 1992, the dance club Renaissance opened in Mansfield where DJs Sasha and John Digweed were instrumental in popularizing its early sound.
  Other notable Progressive House DJs and producers include: Nathan Fake, James Holden, Dave Seaman, Nick Warren, Jason Jollins, Hernan Cattaneo, Deadmau5, Anthony Pappa. Notable active progressive house labels include Baroque Records, Bedrock Records, Renaissance, Audiotherapy, Global Underground and Source of Gravity. **Progressive trance;** is a popular sub-genre in trance music and contains elements of house, techno, and ambient music. By the late 1990s, trance became more focused on the anthemic qualities and melodies, moving away from arpeggiated analog synth patterns. Acoustic elements and spacey pads became popular with compositions leaned towards incremental changes à la progressive structures.

375

Progressive trance contains distinctive sounds in many tracks, such as unusual bass lines or original synthesized sounds, which generally makes it more "catchy". Phrases are usually a power number of bars in most typical progressive trance tracks. Phrases usually begin with the introduction of a new or different melody or rhythm. Compared to trance, the progressive wing is usually deeper and more abstract, featuring a lower average bpm (around 125-135 instead of 130-160) and a recurrent melodic structure. This structure is intuitively described as consisting of three major structural elements: (1) build-up; (2) breakdown; (3) climax. These three structural elements are expressed either temporally or in their intensity, if not both. A 'build-up' sequence can sometimes last up to 3 or even 4 minutes. Subtle incremental/decremental acoustic variations (i.e., gradual addition/subtraction of instruments) anticipate the transition to each subsequent structural element of the track. The initial build-up and the final break-down are generally very similar, adding a feel of symmetry to the general structure of the melody. Furthermore, a progressive trance track is usually longer than a regular trance track, ranging in length from 5-6 to even 12–13 minutes. Although there is a general and increasing tendency to associate progressive trance with progressive house (or vice-versa), virtually rendering these two sub-genres identical, there are however distinctive characteristics apart from the strong similitudes between them: progressive trance inherits from its parent genre (trance) a wider melodic flexibility, while progressive house is usually darker and more minimal. Some of the most representative names that currently work in this sub-genre are Laurent Veronnez, Sasha, Mike Dierickx, Matt Darey, Vibrasphere, Armin Van Buren, Brian Transeau (aka BT), Christopher Lawrence and more recently, Markus Schulz.

91. pg. 276, From Wikipedia: **Theodor Seuss Geisel** (/ˈɡaɪzəl/; March 2, 1904 – September 24, 1991) was an American writer, poet, and cartoonist. He was most widely known for his children's books written and illustrated as **Dr. Seuss**.

He had used the pen name **Dr. Theophrastus Seuss** in college and later used **Theo LeSieg** and **Rosetta Stone**.[2] Geisel published 46 children's books, often characterized by imaginative characters, rhyme, and frequent use of anapestic meter. His most-celebrated books include the bestselling *Green Eggs and Ham*, *The Cat in the Hat*, *The Lorax*, *One Fish Two Fish Red Fish Blue Fish*, *The 500 Hats of Bartholomew Cubbins*, *Fox in Socks*, *The King's Stilts*, *Hop on Pop*, *Thidwick the Big-Hearted Moose*, *Horton Hatches the Egg*, *Horton Hears a Who!*, and *How the Grinch Stole Christmas!*.
His works have spawned numerous adaptations, including 11 television specials, four feature films, a Broadway musical and four television series. He won the Lewis Carroll Shelf Award in 1958 for *Horton Hatches the Egg* and again in 1961 for *And to Think That I Saw It on Mulberry Street*. Geisel also worked as an illustrator for advertising campaigns, most notably for Flit and Standard Oil, and as apolitical cartoonist for *PM*, a New York City newspaper. During World War II, he worked in an animation department of the United States Army, where he wrote *Design for Death*, a film that later won the 1947 Academy Award for Documentary Feature.

He was a perfectionist in his work and would sometimes spend up to a year on a book. It was not uncommon for him to throw out 95% of his material until he settled on a theme for his book. For a writer he was unusual in that he preferred to be paid only after he finished his work rather than in advance.[3] Geisel's birthday, March 2, has been adopted as the annual date for National Read Across America Day, an initiative on reading created by the National Education Association.

92. pg. 277, From Wikipedia: *Horton Hears a Who!* is a children's book written and illustrated by Theodor Seuss Geisel under the name Dr. Seuss and published in 1954 by Random House. It is the second Dr. Seuss book to feature Horton the Elephant, the first being *Horton Hatches the Egg.* The Whos would later make a re-appearance in *How the Grinch Stole Christmas!* Geisel, who had harbored strong anti-Japan sentiments before and during World War II, changed his views dramatically after the war and used this book as an allegory for the American post-war occupation of the country,[1] as well as dedicating the book to a Japanese friend. Plot [edit] The book tells the story of Horton the Elephant, who, in the afternoon of May 15 while splashing in a pool in the Jungle of Nool, hears a small speck of dust talking to him. Horton surmises that a small person lives on the speck and places it on a clover, vowing to protect it. He later discovers that the speck is actually a tiny planet, home to a community called Whoville, where microscopic creatures called Whos live. The Mayor of Whoville asks Horton to protect them from harm, which Horton happily agrees to, proclaiming throughout the book that "a person's a person, no matter how small." In his mission to protect the speck, Horton is ridiculed and harassed by the other animals in the jungle for believing in something that they are unable to see or hear. He is first criticized by a sour kangaroo and the little kangaroo in her pouch. The splash they make as they jump into the pool almost catches the speck, so Horton decides to find somewhere safer for it. However, news of his odd new behavior spreads quickly, and he is soon harassed by the Wickersham Brothers, a group of monkeys. They steal the clover from him and give it to Vlad Vlad-i-koff, an eagle. Vlad-i-koff flies the clover a long distance, Horton in pursuit, until the eagle drops it into a field of clovers. After a long search, Horton finally finds the clover with the speck on it. However, the Mayor informs him that Whoville is in bad shape from the fall, and Horton discovers that the sour kangaroo and the Wickersham family have caught up to him. They tie Horton up and threaten to boil the speck in a pot of "Beezle-Nut" oil. To save Whoville, Horton implores the little people to make as much noise as they can, to prove their existence. So almost everyone in Whoville shouts, sings, and plays instruments, but still no one but Horton can hear them. So the Mayor searches Whoville until he finds a "very small shirker named JoJo", who is playing with a yo-yo instead of making noise. The Mayor carries him to the top of Eiffelberg Tower, where Jojo lets out a loud "Yopp!" which finally makes the kangaroo and the Wickersham family hear the Whos. Now convinced of the Whos's existence, the other jungle animals vow to help Horton protect the tiny community.

93. pg. 280, From Wikipedia: **Om** (written universally as ॐ; in Devanagari as ओं *oṃ* [õ:], ओं *aum* [əʊ], or 'ओ३म्॰ *om* [õ:m]) is a mantra and mystical Sanskrit sound of Hindu origin (geographically India), sacred and important in various Dharmic religions such as Hinduism, Buddhism and Jainism.

The syllable is also referred to as **omkara** (ओंकार *oṃkāra*) or **aumkara** (ओंकार *aumkāra*), literally "om syllable", and in Sanskrit it is sometimes referred to as *pranava*, literally "that which is sounded out loudly". Om is also written ओ३म् (*ōm* [õ::m]), where ३ is *pluta* ("three times as long"), indicating a length of three morae (that is, the time it takes to say three syllables)—an overlong nasalized close-mid back rounded vowel—though there are other enunciations adhered to in received traditions. It is placed at the beginning of most Hindu texts as a sacred incantation to be intoned at the beginning and end of a reading of the Vedas or prior to any prayer or mantra. It is used at the end of the invocation to the god being sacrificed to (*anuvakya*) as an invitation to and for that God to partake of .

94. pg. 280, From Wikipedia: **HU** or **Hu** may refer to: Mythology and religion [edit]

- Hu (mythology), the deification of the first word in the Egyptian mythology of the Ennead
- Huh (god), the deification of eternity in the Egyptian mythology of the Ogdoad
- Hu (Sufism), a name for God
- Hú, a kachina in Hopi mythology
- Adir Hu, a hymn sung at the Passover Seder
- Hu Gadarn, (Hu the Mighty) a Welsh legendary figure
- HU, a mantra popularized by the religion Eckankar as a name for and love song to God   **HU: A Love Song to God;** *HU is woven into the language of life. It is the Sound of all sounds. It is the wind in the leaves, falling rain, thunder of jets, singing of birds, the awful rumble of a tornado. . . . Its sound is heard in laughter, weeping, the din of city traffic, ocean waves, and the quiet rippling of a mountain stream. And yet, the word HU is not God. It is a word people anywhere can use to address the Originator of Life.*

—Harold Klemp

95. pg. 281, From Wikipedia: **Eckankar** is a new religious that focuses on spiritual exercises enabling practitioners to experience what its followers call "the Light and Sound of God." The personal experience of this spiritual Light and Sound is a primary goal of the teaching. It claims to provide a personal, unique and individual spiritual inner path to understanding of self as soul, and development of higher awareness "consciousness" and God. According to the Eckankar glossary, the term *Eckankar* means "Co-Worker with God".[1] It is likely drawn from the Sikh term, Ik Onkar. Since 1985 followers of Eckankar have described it as "The Religion of the Light and Sound of God". Prior to 1985, Eckankar was known as "The Ancient Science of Soul Travel". Eckankar's headquarters are in Chanhassen, Minnesota (southwest of Minneapolis). The Eckankar Temple, an outdoor chapel, an administrative building, and the ECK Spiritual Campus are located at this site.

96. pg. 287, From Wikipedia: **René Descartes** (French: [ʁəne dekaʁt]; Latinized: **Renatus Cartesius**; adjectival form: "Cartesian";[6] 31 March 1596 – 11 February 1650) was a French philosopher, mathematician, and writer who spent most of his life in the Dutch Republic. He has been dubbed *The Father of Modern Philosophy*, and much subsequent Western philosophy is a response to his writings,[7][8] which are studied closely to this day. In particular, his *Meditations on First Philosophy* continues to be a standard text at most university philosophy departments.

Descartes' influence in mathematics is equally apparent; the Cartesian coordinate system — allowing reference to a point in space as a set of numbers, and allowing algebraic equations to be expressed as geometric shapes in a two-dimensional coordinate system (and conversely, shapes to be described as equations) — was named after him. He is credited as the father of analytical geometry, the bridge between algebra and geometry, crucial to the discovery of infinitesimal calculus and analysis. Descartes was also one of the key figures in the Scientific Revolution and has been described as an example of genius. He refused to accept the authority of previous philosophers and also refused to accept the obviousness of his own senses. Descartes frequently sets his views apart from those of his predecessors. In the opening section of the *Passions of the Soul*, a treatise on the Early Modern version of what are now commonly called emotions, Descartes goes so far as to assert that he will write on this topic "as if no one had written on these matters before". Many elements of his philosophy have precedents in late Aristotelianism, the revived Stoicism of the 16th century, or in earlier philosophers like Augustine.

In his natural philosophy, he differs from the schools on two major points: First, he rejects the splitting of corporeal substance into matter and form; second, he rejects any appeal to final ends—divine or natural—in explaining natural phenomena.[9] In his theology, he insists on the absolute freedom of God's act of creation. Descartes laid the foundation for 17th-century continental rationalism, later advocated by Baruch Spinoza and Gottfried Leibniz, and opposed by the empiricist school of thought consisting of Hobbes, Locke, Berkeley, Jean-Jacques Rousseau, and Hume. Leibniz, Spinoza and Descartes were all well versed in mathematics as well as philosophy, and Descartes and Leibniz contributed greatly to science as well. He is perhaps best known for the philosophical statement "*Cogito ergo sum*" (French: *Je pense, donc je suis*; English: I think, therefore I am), found in part IV of *Discourse on the Method* (1637 – written in French but with inclusion of "*Cogito ergo sum*") and §7 of part I of *Principles of Philosophy*(1644 – written in Latin).

97. pg. 256, *Machaneers:* A term used to define those *functioning* as *cause.* A *machaneer* is a master engineer of *process* or *causation mechanics.* This represents a functional capacity to *be unconditional,* as a channel or conduit of *source,* using *USL; universal sound language,* through the *clockwise spiral out-flow* and the *counter-clockwise spiral in-flow,* linked to all *fascial membrane frequencies,* both physical and non-physical, to *create* and *manifest* the figure eight *mobius* of *infinity* into the *double helix* of the *toroidal sphere,* to travel through the *singularities* of *black holes,* to *wake-up, remember* and *transcend STEM; space-time,* energy and matter. To *be a co-worker* with the *divine.* This term was shared directly to me by a *machaneer* at a sacred *USL* gathering.

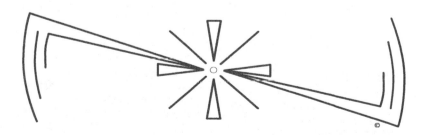

INDEX

Symbols

A

M

magic, 45, 176, 209, 239, 365, 367

Magic Penny, 209, 365, *See Malvina Reynolds, See* songs

magnetic, 6, 95, 96, 211, 229, 252, 254, 255, 259, 260, 262, 272, 274, 284, 318, 324, 351, See shifting, See poles

magnetic poles, 252, 254, 255, 259, 260, 262, 272, 284

magnetism, 230, 231, 259, 292, 319

magnetosphere, 230

magnification, 60, 67, 68, 69, 70, 71, 72, 73, 74, 75, 76, 77, 78, 79, 80, 81, 127, 325

Mahayuga, 310, *See* One day in the life of Brahma, *See* Hindu cycle of cosmic history, Satya, Tretya, Dwapara and Kali yugas

male dominant, 255

Malvina Reynolds, 209, 365, *See* Magic Penny

Man, 206, 220, 221, 235, 273, 275, 276, 374

mandala, 57

mandate, 43, 45, 222, 225, 243

Mandelbrot Set, 65, 66, 83

manifest, 11, 38, 51, 53, 60, 62, 63, 66, 83, 100, 102, 119, 129, 141, 147, 157, 162, 164, 165, 167, 168, 169, 172, 201, 206, 215, 216, 221, 223, 224, 232, 239, 241, 242, 244, 247, 253, 277, 279, 280, 282, 285, 286, 287, 288, 289, 290, 291, 315, 327, 328, 340, 379, *See* things

manifestation, 32, 33, 34, 55, 60, 63, 66, 83, 99, 122, 132, 144, 147, 150, 165, 169, 199, 206, 214, 216, 223, 225, 238, 242, 254, 255, 262, 285, 349

mantra, 55, 100, 102, 104, 159, 195, 235, 262, 279, 283, 326, 377, 378, *See* USL

Marcus Bach, 194, *See* The Inner Ecstasy

martial artist, 175, 362, *See* Bruce Lee

massage, 118, 334, 354, 358, 360

master, 29, 37, 118, 175, 176, 177, 189, 195, 225, 245, 248, 351, 361, 363

mathematical, 39, 40, 51, 52, 130, 142, 156, 284, 286, 291, 292

mathematician, 65, 117, 350, 352, 378

Mathematics, 3, 38, 39, *See* pure universal language

matriarchal, 255, 263, *See* female, Earth mother

matrix, 51, 52, 55, 192, 201, 205, 221, 268, 270, 271, 276

matter, 4, 12, 53, 126, 127, 128, 129, 130, 143, 164, 165, 170, 171, 231, 283, 285, 286, 288, 289, 290, 327, 348, 352, 370, 377, 379, *See* empty space

Matter is mostly Empty Space, 4, 129

Matthew 6:24-33, 166, *See* bible

Mayan Calendar, 250, 252, 272

Mayan numerical system, 40, *See* base 20

Mayan Tree of Life, 280

mechanics, 32, 204, 379

mechanics of causation, 131, 133, *See* causation mechanics

mechanisms, 44, 94, 371

medicine, 5, 10, 93, 108, 143, 161, 167, 224, 230, 234, 235, 348, 353, 354, 356, 358, 360, 371

meditation, 90, 104, 179, 235, 254, 341, 348, 367, 372, *See* contemplation

medium, 18, 32, 39, 56, 63, 98, 103, 112, 116, 140, 146, 154, 162, 166, 188, 193, 242, 244, 278, 362

membrane, 4, 5, 6, 11, 17, 18, 29, 36, 37, 48, 49, 50, 51, 53, 54, 57, 60, 62, 63, 65, 66, 83, 84, 88, 89, 99, 101, 102, 103, 111, 112, 114, 115, 119, 125, 129, 143, 146, 147, 157, 179, 181, 185, 188, 190, 199, 200,

400

405

CPSIA information can be obtained
at www.ICGtesting.com
Printed in the USA
FSOW03n1524251016
26543FS